Palliative Care
in the Acute
Hospital Setting:
A Practical Guide

Palliative Care in the Acute Hospital Setting: A Practical Guide

Sara Booth
Macmillan Consultant in Palliative Medicine
Director Palliative Care Services
Addenbrookes NHS Trust

Polly Edmonds
Consultant in Palliative Medicine
Palliative Care Team
King's College Hospital NHS Foundation Trust

Margaret Kendall
Macmillan Consultant Nurse in Palliative Care
Delamere Centre
Warrington and Halton Hospitals NHS Foundation Trust

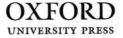

OXFORD
UNIVERSITY PRESS

OXFORD
UNIVERSITY PRESS

Great Clarendon Street, Oxford OX2 6DP

Oxford University Press is a department of the University of Oxford.
It furthers the University's objective of excellence in research, scholarship,
and education by publishing worldwide in

Oxford New York

Auckland Cape Town Dar es Salaam Hong Kong Karachi
Kuala Lumpur Madrid Melbourne Mexico City Nairobi
New Delhi Shanghai Taipei Toronto

With offices in

Argentina Austria Brazil Chile Czech Republic France Greece
Guatemala Hungary Italy Japan Poland Portugal Singapore
South Korea Switzerland Thailand Turkey Ukraine Vietnam

Oxford is a registered trade mark of Oxford University Press
in the UK and in certain other countries

Published in the United States
by Oxford University Press Inc., New York

British Library Cataloguing in Publication Data
Data available

Library of Congress Cataloging in Publication Data
Data available

Typeset by Cepha Imaging Pvt. Ltd., Bangalore
Printed in Great Britain
on acid-free paper by the
MPG Books Group, Bodmin and King's Lynn

ISBN 978–0–19–923892–7 (pbk)

1 3 5 7 9 10 8 6 4 2

Preface

The majority of people in the UK spend time in hospital in the last year of their life and will die there, yet palliative care is still associated in many people's minds (both clinicians and general public) solely with hospices and care-giving charities and with caring for people with cancer. However, most people with palliative care needs have non-malignant disease and are seen and treated by acute hospital services; there is increasing acceptance and recognition that these groups have not received equitable access to the specialty. It is also accepted widely that what has loosely been called 'supportive care' needs to be integrated with palliative care so that the end-of-life problems of symptom control and psychosocial distress for people with any life-threatening or life-limiting illness can be prevented rather than heroically treated. To accomplish these aims palliative care services need to see patients during hospital attendances or admissions, which may be at the time of diagnosis of a life-threatening or -limiting condition during an acute exacerbation, during treatment, or at the end of life.

This book aims to help palliative care clinicians set up, continue to develop, and run an effective service for the acute hospital setting. It is aimed specifically at senior clinicians undertaking management roles and responsibilities but will also be useful to doctors, nurses, and therapists who are training or developing and likely to undertake more senior roles in the future – or to better understand the context in which they are working. The book has been written by three clinicians who have worked in hospital palliative care for over 10 years and been part of the development of these services. It is written to be used a practical manual as the reader chooses (either dip into a relevant chapter or read from cover to cover) and describes some of the skills and attributes useful in such services, in addition to reviewing important basic knowledge. This book is not intended to be a textbook of Palliative Care – instead it is to be used alongside such books to support clinicians in developing acute hospital palliative care services.

The topics covered in this book are those which we think are central to operating in the acute hospital environment, which is so very different in scope and culture from the hospice or community setting. Chapter 1 reviews these differences with a view to limiting the potential mistake of making continual comparisons with hospice care and finding the hospital wanting. We recognize that some clinicians are in the hospital because of the need to provide support to a hospital palliative care team (e.g. a consultant from a local hospice) or from rotation or placement, and not as their first choice – if this is your situation, we would recommend that you start with Chapter 1 – it will help smooth your transition into hospital palliative care.

Chapter 2 considers the structure and function of the team. A stand-alone multi-professional hospital team is becoming the norm now (or at least an outreach service from a local hospice or specialist palliative care team). As health services across the world moves to 'payment by procedure' with an increasing focus on income generation, it is important to remember the roots of hospital palliative care and continue to promote the quality agenda. We hope that this chapter facilitates this.

Chapter 3 gives tips and ideas on organizing clinical care – based on our experience in these services. It is essential for credibility in the acute hospital setting to be accessible and flexible as well as competent with well-honed specialist skills. Fluctuating demand can make organization tricky and Chapter 3 will help consider this and will be useful to both newly formed teams and those that are looking to develop further.

Chapter 4 is concerned with becoming embedded in the hospital; not an 'optional add-on' service when money can be found or an extraneous visitation. Palliative care needs to be a core activity of the hospital (like radiology or pathology) and be flexible enough to respond to demand. In this chapter we consider how hospital palliative care teams, mainly working in an advisory capacity, can consider how they demonstrate their 'added value' and meet their own and Trusts' clinical governance agendas.

Chapter 5 covers the essential topic of support for team members – keeping up the momentum for changes in development in the Trust without taking a toll on individual clinicians within palliative care service.

Chapter 6 helps you to understand the principles of bureaucracy and money – key for palliative care services which are often funded from a variety of sources, both charitable and governmental.

Education, research, and audit are covered in some depth in subsequent chapters, leading to a final chapter on personal development and support. We believe that all of these issues are central to increasing our knowledge base and expanding understanding of how to practice our specialty and to increase its expertise, so that no patient or family is denied access to it by ignorance. Some suggestions for personal survival are outlined in Chapter 10 – this work is to be enjoyed, but it can sometimes be overshadowed by the demands of giving excellent palliative care in the acute, fast-moving, competitive Trust.

We hope that this book will provide a useful resource to clinicians practising in the acute setting. It is not meant to be the answer to everything but to give a structure, support, and ideas for clinicians to set up and develop their services as we all strive for delivering excellent palliative care in the challenging acute setting.

Dr Sara Booth
Dr Polly Edmonds
Mrs Margaret Kendall
May 2009

Contents

Chapter 1

Palliative care in the acute hospital

Why have you chosen to work in an acute hospital?

If you are reading this book, it is because you are, or you are thinking of, working in an acute setting as well as or instead of a hospice. What drew you to this setting? Was it the excitement, the ever-changing pattern of working, the interaction with colleagues from many other disciplines, and the almost limitless potential for applying palliative care principles to people with a wide range of acute and chronic illnesses? You may, of course, be working in a hospice and keen to extend your service to the local hospital – or be asked to and need to make a start. It is important to have some idea what you are taking on in an acute setting, where the culture of the acute Trust is very different from a hospice and your work practices need to be tailored to this environment.

Acute hospitals are geared to managing short-term, sudden onset illnesses: getting people over either a time-limited health crisis or an episode or exacerbation in a long-term illness. Despite this, long-lasting poor health and chronic disease are the major health problems of the twenty-first century and dying is something that is common to all of us. Hospitals are not really set up to deal with either situation as their roots and systems of operation derive from centuries ago. Most of the staff working in acute hospitals will not have had any training in palliative care. That will change over time as clinicians coming through nursing and medical school have had exposure to palliative care teaching which is also becoming embedded in the training of allied healthcare professionals, pharmacists, and others working in clinical roles. We are some way from that happy situation at the moment.

In a hospice everyone in that institution will be working towards promoting excellent palliative care. They are all committed to it, at least for the time they work there; volunteers, chief executives, fundraisers, as well as the doctors and nurses will all understand the basic ideals of palliative care to a greater or lesser extent. Palliative care will be central to their working identity and what they measure themselves by every day. In a large teaching hospital, where there might be around 1000 beds, perhaps 15 people (at most) will be palliative care specialists. Many of the clinicians and others working in the hospital will actually actively want to avoid or minimize their contact with palliative care issues as they would see themselves as training in medicine or nursing or management or basic science primarily to save lives.

Qualities that will help you thrive in the acute hospital

There are no absolute rights or wrongs, but some personal qualities are particularly important if you are to thrive and survive in an acute hospital:

1. You must be able to live with imperfection: you are probably going to achieve 60% of ideal palliative care rather than 95% as you might be in a hospice.
2. Enthusiasm for being in the hospital is a must: you must like the atmosphere and feel attuned to the way it works.
3. You must like working alongside other specialists and not feel they are heartless technocrats.
4. You must be able to withstand discouragement and slow bureaucracy.
5. You must not take it personally or be downhearted when the Trust or other clinicians in it have different priorities for you.
6. Resilience and the ability to persist in putting forward your ideas are key qualities.
7. You need to be able to take a 'long view', as your ideas may take some time to come to fruition.
8. You must believe passionately in the idea of palliative care in the acute setting.
9. You need to be able to work in a relatively small team – at times this can be an intense experience, but you need to be able to work like this.
10. You need to be able to live with being a 'small fish in a big pond' and to work in an environment where not everyone understands what you do in a context of competing priorities, rather than palliative care being the sole function of the organization.

Acute palliative care

Palliative care in the acute setting needs to be flexible and responsive to best integrate into the hospital. Most hospital palliative care teams see a relatively higher proportion of non-cancer patients with long-term conditions than hospice or community services and have the advantage of having the 'experts' on hand, so a model of shared care can be more realistic. In addition, in the acute

Case study: Palliative care and haematology

Traditionally, palliative care teams and haematologists have not always had the most constructive or easy working relationships. In one of our organizations an opportunity arose for a member of the palliative care team (initially an interested specialist registrar; now a consultant) to attend the weekly haemato-oncology ward round. Over the years, this interaction has led to an increased understanding of the skills that each specialty group can offer and has led not only to a marked increase in referrals (the second largest cancer referral group in our organization), but also to the palliative care team, managing the acute symptom control on the haemato-oncology and bone marrow transplant units.

Patients having treatment with curative intent are now regularly referred for management of nausea and vomiting, painful mucositis, diarrhoea, and other troublesome symptoms; and the team's psychosocial worker works alongside the haemato-oncology nurse specialists and counsellor to provide specialist welfare benefits advice and support to patients and families, including young children.

One positive outcome of this interaction, that is now well embedded into the culture of the unit, is that it is incredibly rare to be told that 'they're not ready for you yet' (which used to be a common occurrence) and the palliative care team are commonly involved in discussions regarding advance care planning for those patients with progressive disease or for those who are dying from the complications of treatment.

setting many teams will see patients when they are still having treatment with curative intent (see case study) – or whilst they are in the process of being investigated for potentially life-threatening or life-limiting illnesses (see case study) – so a much larger proportion of patients that will survive. This should not be a problem and fits with a model of acute or short-term interventions from palliative care that characterizes palliative care in the acute setting.

The key to successfully developing your service and your own skills is to become adept at transferring your generic palliative care skills into the acute setting. You may have to be pragmatic (in what you can achieve), you will certainly have to be flexible, and you may need to be creative and/or imaginative. Be prepared for a high turnover of patients, of not owning the patients when working in an advisory role, and of a need to do what you can do within the confines of the acute setting. You will also need to ensure that you have systems to enable excellent communication with hospice and community colleagues as you will often have to handover patients whose problems and issues are 'work in progress'.

Case study: Palliative care and neurology

Two of us work in acute Trusts with tertiary neurology services. Following some specific service development to promote palliative care in neurology in one of our organizations, referrals have increased and can now be for acute symptom control or for specialist psychosocial support, even in people without a formal diagnosis. In several of these situations patients' symptoms have been adequately controlled prior to a clear diagnosis or clinical improvement being confirmed – but once the 'acute' palliative care problems have been resolved, the patients can be discharged from palliative care. It can be reassuring for teams in the acute setting to see that interventions from palliative care do not harm the patient and can be positively received both by patients and families.

Being successful in the acute hospital setting

Whilst there are no absolute rights and wrongs to successfully developing hospital palliative care teams, strong clinical leadership and a cohesive sense of team are crucial. These issues are expanded on and discussed in more detail throughout the book, but here we discuss some aspects of teamwork that we feel are vitally important.

Developing a sense of 'team'

People may choose careers in Palliative Care with widely differing expectations and motivations but for teams to function effectively, some agreed shared vision and objectives are crucial and can help to engender team spirit and identity. As most hospital palliative care staff will be working in an advisory setting in the acute hospital, a sense of shared team identity when out and about on the wards can be supportive and empowering, whatever people's professional backgrounds. So in any service, whether new or established, it can be useful to spend some time in a team meeting or Away Day, considering a shared vision for the team or service that helps to foster team spirit and a sense of meaning and belonging for team members. Time invested in understanding team members' motivation for choosing to work in a hospital palliative care team can also be useful and can help senior clinicians understand how and why staff react to certain situations or challenges in certain ways. Whilst it is unrealistic to expect everyone to have the same degree of motivation and enthusiasm, understanding what drew team members to this team at this point in time may enable you as a senior clinician or team leader to draw out the best in them.

In addition, flexibility is crucial to ensuring that any team works well and achieves its objectives. When a team is being set up from the outset, no precedents have been set and working practices can be flexible to meet the needs of the team and service. Even in established teams, when there are team changes and new members are being appointed, it is a golden opportunity to examine whether better productivity and, perhaps more importantly, greater professional satisfaction can be achieved by making changes.

Supporting the team

Adequate support between team members is also a vital component of good team dynamics. It can be helpful for team members to meet together at least once a day; some meet at either end of the day. This gives a good opportunity to discuss the case load, facilitate clinical prioritization, and to feedback on difficult patients, families, or teams (see Chapter 4 for more detail). Talking through how difficult situations could be managed may put a different perspective on a problem; equally a debriefing session after a difficult situation can be very supportive and facilitate shared learning. In the longer term, such informal support can make the difference between being able to cope well with the rigours of the post and stress levels escalating, which can then lead to sick leave.

Regular supervision meetings between team members and their line managers can be supportive and can facilitate early airing of any problems or issues. In practice individual team members are unlikely to want to share worries or concerns in a larger group setting such as a team meeting, but may raise issues in a one-to-one meeting. There are no fixed rules as to the structure or content of such meetings, but we have found more informal meetings as often as weekly in between more formal appraisal, assessment, or performance review meetings to be helpful and supportive for managers and team members alike.

What's in a name?

One issue in the acute setting can be how your team are known. Many people either do not know what palliative care is or associate it purely with end-of-life care. Some people argue that the terminology 'Palliative Care' can be a barrier in the acute hospital – particularly if your team are seeing people who are having curative treatment; in this context some teams will call themselves the Supportive Care Team. The authors all work in teams that see a wide variety of patients, including those receiving curative treatment – and use the term Hospital Palliative Care Team. In our experience this has rarely been problematic and when it is, this is usually more of an issue for staff rather than for patients or families. What seems more important to us is that you are clear about what skills your team have to offer, that you get out and about and that you demonstrate your value by good clinical outcomes. As an example, referring to Case study 1, in the acute haematology, the ward team will usually inform patients and families of the referral to palliative care and the Palliative Care Team then introduce themselves as such. In our experience, this is not easily an issue and our concern is that moving to the term Supportive Care Team may be confusing and not adequately reflect the team's skills and expertise – but the ultimate decisions need to be dictated by what is right for a specific organization.

Starting out as a consultant or nurse specialist

The transition from a specialist registrar to medical consultant, from nurse specialist to nurse consultant, or from a ward or community nurse to a clinical nurse specialist can be very challenging and take people well outside of their comfort zone.

Case study: First year as a consultant

Ahmed had significant experience in oncology before he started training in palliative medicine: he had changed specialty because he was less interested in oncological treatments than in symptom control and was keen to have more time to talk to patients than was allocated in oncology clinics. After starting at the Royal Western (a tertiary referral centre), he became exhausted within his first year as he felt – as he put it, 'everyone wants a slice' – he was expected to be at every MDT, PCT, oncology network meeting, as well as in dealing with significant interpersonal issues within the team. He felt guilty that he rarely saw a patient. His clinical director, an oncologist, did not understand Ahmed's job plan. He was late home on many evenings and snappy and unkind when he was there. He started to think he had made a terrible mistake – so did his family. The tide turned after he returned from a conference where he met a previous educational adviser who gave him some tips about time management, prioritizing, remembering that his career would most usefully be a marathon not a sprint. She offered telephone mentoring to help him sort out a manageable way of doing his job. A year later, life was better, he felt fitter, and his home life was happier although the bureaucracy remained unchanged.

For many doctors by the time they complete their registrar training and achieve their certificate of completion of training, they will feel ready and able to step up into a consultant post. However, even for the most confident doctor, the transition to consultant can be similar to that of medical student to junior doctor – you have the theory but the reality can be isolating and extremely stressful. Consultant posts can be isolated – you may be the only consultant on the team and, if lead clinician, will take ultimate responsibility for the team's performance. In the move from registrar to consultant you also lose your immediate peer group – and it can take time to find your feet and join a new one. This is exacerbated working in an acute hospital setting where you are usually not part of an established consultant team – therefore from day 1 you will have to take responsibility across the board – not just for clinical activity, but also for governance, teaching, training, and management. In your enthusiasm to impress it is easy to take on too much too soon – we would strongly advise you to seek advice and support from a more experienced consultant in your area, so that you do not find yourself out of your depth and with too much to do within months. Many acute hospital Trusts also run management development programmes for new consultants – these are helpful not only in developing your knowledge and skills, but also in finding a peer group within the organization. You will find more detail regarding 'surviving as a senior clinician' in palliative care in Chapter 10.

Chapter 2

Getting started: structure and function of the team

The first hospital palliative care team in the UK was started by Dr. Thelma Bates in 1977. Dr. Bates was a consultant clinical oncologist at St. Thomas' Hospital in London, who had worked closely with Dame Cicely Saunders at St. Christopher's Hospice. Her aim was to take the excellence of palliative care from hospices back into the acute setting. The need for hospital palliative care teams has increasingly been recognized so that in the UK alone, in 2008, there are over 250 such teams.

In the early days of specialist palliative care in hospitals and before the development of palliative care as a separate specialty, a support team often developed almost by default. There may have been an experienced ward nurse or senior doctor who had a particular leaning towards palliative care on his/her ward and a body of expertise developed within one area. This same person may have been called upon to give advice to other ward areas. Gradually hospital management teams may have created a niche post for that particular person and renamed them as a specialist nurse or consultant with a special interest. Those days are long gone, with a need to justify the added value of any new posts, which are often 'target-driven'. However, the 2004 NICE 'Improving Outcomes Guidance for Supportive and Palliative Care' did help to define the make-up of a hospital palliative care team, and this has supported team development in some places. The report by the National Council for Palliative Care, 'Palliative Care 2000: Commissioning through Partnership', also gave guidance on the numbers of team members required in an acute Trust, but this information should only be regarded as guidance and more recent service reconfigurations mean that its guidance is probably outdated.

The hospital palliative care team

Who do you need in the hospital palliative care team?

The 2004 Manual for Cancer Services outlined the standard for personnel in a hospital palliative care team, its recommendations based on the NICE

Improving Outcomes guidance. This recommended that the team is made up of two elements: a core team and an extended team.

The core team

As a minimum, this consists of

1. Palliative medicine specialist
2. Palliative care nurse specialist
3. Multi-disciplinary team (MDT) co-ordinator/secretary

Within several teams in the country, there are now also Palliative Care Consultant nurses, who will fulfil a very different function to that of the specialist nurse as outlined in Table 1.1 below. You need to think what works best in your Trust e.g. if consultant nurses are appointed to outreach roles (such as ITU) would this be an effective way for your team to work?

Table 1.1 Differences between nurse specialists and consultant nurses

Roles undertaken	Consultant nurse	Clinical nurse specialist	Advantage to palliative care service
Managerial role	Sometimes	Occasionally as team leader	Consultant needs to be politically astute and can bring about change management by operational and strategic working
Autonomous clinical role	Has considerable experience in a senior level in palliative care often with a minimum of 10 years clinical experience	Needs to have the ability to work as an autonomous practitioner, and has at least 5 years post basic experience	Consultant could set up specialist service, e.g. breathlessness or hold clinics independent of medical practitioner
Research	Leads and conducts research	Demonstrates awareness of, and uses research to underpin practice	Consultant often has academic position as an integral part of the role, forging good links with higher educational institute (HEIs) to influence and assist in curriculum development
Practice development	Involved in national policy development	Involved in local +/− network policy development	Ability to influence local and national policy by representation of palliative care services at a strategic level

Table 1.1 (continued) Differences between nurse specialists and consultant nurses

Roles undertaken	Consultant nurse	Clinical nurse specialist	Advantage to palliative care service
Cross boundary working	May provide clinical care across all care settings	Usually practicses in one specific area	Able to influence service development in all areas by liaison with commissioning bodies
Education	Provides education up to and including Masters level.	Delivers education within own sphere of practice	Ensures palliative care education is firmly embedded into pro-grammes of nursing and medical training. Provides supervision and mentorship for trainees and newly appointed staff
Clinical governance	Usually has responsibility up to Board level	Responsible for local governance	Consultant has ability to influence charge at highest level

The extended team

The extended team can include any or all of the following:

1. Clinical psychologist
2. Social worker
3. At least one person agreed as representing care for patients' and carers' rehabilitation needs, e.g. occupational or physiotherapist
4. At least one person agreed as representing care for patients' and carers' spiritual needs (in most, but not all cases represented by a person from chaplaincy)
5. At least one person agreed as representing bereavement care for families and carers
6. Oncologist
7. Anaesthetist with interest in pain; expertise in nerve blocking and neuro-modulation techniques
8. Pharmacist

Further members of a specialist palliative care multi-disciplinary team (MDT) have been recommended by NICE to also include:

1. Dietician
2. Speech and language therapist

3. Providers of complementary therapy

4. Providers of creative activity/art therapists, etc.

Very few hospital palliative care teams have large extended teams; even today, some teams consist only of a doctor and nurses, or even only one of these professions. Uni-professional teams do not meet current guidance, cannot be considered multi-professional, and are no longer encouraged.

In practice, there are usually more nurses on hospital palliative care teams than other team members and once a critical mass is reached, some teams decide to go down the route of appointing a nursing team leader. It may well be that this is at a later stage of team development, with the 'leader' being chosen from within the existing team, in order to develop and support the nursing team effectively. For teams 'in trouble' it may be a management decision that brings about the creation of this role.

Sometimes it is preferable to appoint nursing or medical leaders from outside the current establishment, as it is sometimes hard to move into a management role within the same team, particularly if the appointment is taking place because of difficulties within the team. Senior appointments from outside also facilitate a cross-fertilization of ideas across organizations, which is healthy.

There is no defined way to set up a hospital team; it is often a process of evolution, with the most important aspect being developing a team that works well together for a common purpose.

Most hospitals in the UK now have some form of palliative care team, so setting up a team from scratch is unusual. In this situation, however, it is important that some form of needs assessment is undertaken in order to inform service development.

Setting up a new team or developing an established team

Whether starting a new team or developing an established team, there are several factors to consider:

1. The composition of the team.

   i. What is the optimum team structure to meet the needs of the acute Trust?

   ii. How are other advisory teams (e.g. liaison psychiatry) structured in your Trust?

   iii. How many members will the team consist of?

   iv. What is the appropriate professional mix?

   v. Does the team meet NICE standards?

2. How will the team be managed?

    i. Would it be beneficial to have a nursing team leader from the outset, and if so, what would be the benefits of this leader to the team?

    ii. Who will be the clinical lead? (This does not necessarily have to be a medical consultant.)

3. How will the team function?

    i. Will all team members be full time or is the team able to support flexible working?

    ii. Can the team support seven day a week visiting and out of hours provision?

4. What are the competencies required to support the delivery of specialist palliative care in the Trust?

    i. Do existing team members have these competencies, and if not, what training is available to support their development?

5. The local context of specialist palliative care provision into which the hospital team will fit or develop:

    i. What others services are available locally for the provision of Specialist Palliative Care?

    ii. How would a new or improved service impact/interface with existing services?

Team structures

There is no ideal team structure, and certainly not one size fits all; all the authors of this book work within different team structures, many of which have evolved over time. Whatever team structure you are in when you are recruiting new personnel, one of the criteria should be whether they can fit in the existing team. Clearly the team needs to be housed together whatever local management structures prevail – for example it is still common for medical input to be provided and paid for by a neighbouring hospice and the nurses to be managed separately within the hospital hierarchy.

Most hospital services will have a lead clinician for palliative care. One challenge is to ensure that adequate management structures are in place to enable the team to be supported and effectively developed as one unit. In practice only larger teams have a nursing team leader of a different banding; this can lead to problems in smaller teams, as very often the nurse specialists are managed by a nurse who has no background or understanding of palliative care.

This important topic is discussed in more detail in the section, 'Management of the team' (see below).

Accommodation

The integrated team structure, where community and hospital staffs are housed together, often works extremely well, and is lauded in some areas as the ideal. Communication issues are reduced because it is easier to have better liaison when staff are sited together. Logistically though this may be difficult to achieve, as office space is often at a premium.

Suitable accommodation for the entire team is vital for effective working. Having the whole team housed together, providing there are adequate resources, can enhance good communication. The principle of 'hot desking', which is becoming more prevalent in the modern National Health Service (NHS), does not lend itself to cohesive working within a stressful specialty. Equally vital is administrative support. Many key tasks can be undertaken by a good secretarial staff, for example receipt and logging of referrals, maintaining databases of patients, collation of statistics, and preparation of data for MDT meetings. A good secretary can be the lynchpin of the team; however, the recruitment of this key member should ensure they also have access to debriefing and supervision, as they may be the first contact with distressed patients or relatives ringing for advice. A robust IT system should be in place to support the team. An integrated IT system where all health care professionals can access up- to- date information on a patient is the ideal. This is especially useful where out of hours (OOH) working is incorporated into the team rota and staff can access entries by other health care professionals to a patient record.

Management of the team

The management structures of hospital palliative care teams are varied, but if you are new to an existing team or involved in setting one up, this is *one of the most important decisions that has to be made*.

Palliative care in trust management structures

Most hospital teams are managed by acute hospital NHS Trusts; in some circumstances they are, however, managed by Primary Care Trusts (PCTs), effectively providing 'in-reach' to the acute Trust. Whilst there are cogent arguments, e.g. promotion of continuity of care, for hospital and community teams to be managed as one unit, in practice this can pose significant challenges. Acute hospital managers may have little understanding of the delivery of palliative care in the community and managers in PCTs may have limited knowledge of the role of a hospital palliative care team. Such difficulties can affect service development – there are, however, many examples of community and hospital teams thriving under one management structure and you need to appraise local conditions when making these decisions.

A word of warning: management arrangements are frequently re- organized and the individuals in management positions stay a relatively short time in one job. In a well functioning team, if a significant change occurs in the management structure, this may result in the team losing management support, which can significantly affect day to day working. In a worst case scenario, management changes may lead to the team being, 're-positioned' or nursing staff 're-deployed' to help meet the targets in another specialty (particularly in the PCTs), and your effectiveness in the Trust is rapidly lost. Always keep the 'core' aims of hospital palliative care in mind (and keep reminding others of them) when considering where the palliative care team for the Trust should be placed. PCTs will often think that specialist palliative can be done more cheaply by other generalists: if the hospital support team is lost, there will be no other team in the hospital doing the same job. You must be vigilant about the potential consequences of management change.

Where hospital palliative care teams are managed within acute Trusts, they are often considered part of oncology services either in an Oncology Division or within Medicine (or Specialist Medicine for one of the authors). Being closely associated with oncology has clear historical links and also reflects the referral base for many services. One risk of this, however, is that palliative care comes to be seen as synonymous with cancer and this may limit referrals for patients with diagnoses other than cancer. In order to get round this risk clear referral criteria, based on need rather than diagnosis, are required and opportunities sought to promote the fact that palliative care should be considered for all people with life-limiting illnesses. Such opportunities are discussed in more detail in Chapter 4 (being part of the mainstream). In our experience, being managed under the auspices of oncology or medicine is not in itself problematic – what is required for effective service delivery and development is building working relationships within the Division and across the Trust to ensure ongoing managerial support for your service.

Most acute hospitals are divided into Divisions or directorates for management purposes; each will have a general manager, clinical director (usually a senior consultant), senior nurse, and then business and service managers supporting the senior staff. Depending on the size of the Trust, the medical consultant may be professionally and managerially accountable to the clinical director or to another senior clinician. The nurses may be directly responsible to the senior nurse of the Division or, if there is a lead nurse on the team, he/ she will manage the other nurses but be accountable to the Division's Head of Nursing. Management structures vary between organizations – what is crucial is that you understand the structures within your own team. Many Trusts will appoint a lead clinician of the palliative care team, who is likely to be either a medical or nurse consultant; the lead clinician is the organizational face of the service and will represent palliative care across the Trust and at key meetings, such as Division meetings and Trust cancer meetings (see Chapter 6 – for more detail).

In practice the management structures of NHS organizations means that even if a hospital palliative care team has a lead clinician, each professional group is likely to have its own line management structure. So the nurses will be managed by senior nurses and the doctors by senior doctors. In large teams with several members of the same professional groups, a lead nurse may manage all the nurse specialists and potentially other non-medical staff, such as a palliative care social worker; the senior medical consultant is likely to manage all the other doctors on the team. In small teams, with perhaps only one doctor, one or two nurses, and an administrator, it is possible for all team members to be managed by different personnel. Such differences in line management can cause tensions in palliative care teams and it also means that team members may be managed by professionals who have never worked in palliative care and may have a limited understanding of the role(s). In these situations, it may be important to invite members of the management team to spend some time with the team, in order to see palliative care in practice and gain a better understanding of the role(s). Another way to ensure that objectives from individuals' appraisals are linked to the needs of the palliative care service is to organize joint appraisal. For example, the work of the PA to a palliative care consultant is unlikely to be similar to many other secretaries in the oncology department (who will have many more patient letters to write) and appraisal solely by a manager outside palliative care may be unhelpful. If the PA has problems, the manager outside may not be able to understand them. Conversely, it is essential for everyone to have a manager in their profession and outside the team as well who can give another perspective and keep them in line with what is reasonable.

In time you will probably need a 'senior management team' within the palliative care service itself: this might comprise the lead nurse, lead consultant, and psychologist, for example. The lead manager for your division or directorate could also come to the team management meetings: (i) he/she will get a better understanding of what you are trying to achieve and of difficulties intrinsic to driving team strategy forward and (ii) more than any other specialty, palliative care support teams cannot develop separately from the general thrust of the hospital's development, as most work as consultation services and therefore are linked inextricably with other specialities.

If you are working in an AHSC (Academic Health Science Centre), do ensure that you are involved and engaged in discussions around developing partnerships: these may help to develop your service as well as any research you are involved with.

Managing a palliative care service

In managing a successful service it is important to build a framework for meetings into the calendar in order to inform and involve team members of key issues both within the organization and in your locality (or nationally if relevant). You should consider meetings that cover:

1. Team Business
2. Clinical governance, including risk management and audit
3. CPD, e.g. journal club alternating perhaps with team teaching given by different team members and outside speakers from other teams in the hospital
4. If relevant for your service, you may also want to consider meetings covering research and or development
5. Senior management meetings for larger services (as discussed earlier)

We have found it useful for meetings to be scheduled regularly so that they become routine, and it may be appropriate to consider rotation of the chair with all team members then taking some responsibility, as chair, for the meeting content, for the smooth running of the meeting, and the checking of minutes. This gives good experience to team members and limits the meeting becoming dominated by one or a few key individuals with other team members becoming disengaged.

It is also worth considering an annual Away Day when the focus is more strategic; these may be combined with team building sessions (see Chapters 5 and 6 for more consideration of this).

Operational policies

Any palliative care service should have their key clinical operational issues outlined in an operational policy; the requirement for such a document is highlighted in the *Manual for Cancer Service Standards*. Key issues that should be covered in an operational policy if writing or updating one are:

1. Date of policy and review date
2. Mission statement
3. Core and extended team members details
4. Scope of the service and operational detail
   i. Referral criteria
   ii. Referral processes

    iii. Managing workload

    iv. MDMs

    v. Discharge criteria

    vi. Out of hours and 7 day a week working

    vii. Dependency scores/outcome measures (if appropriate)

    viii. Bereavement follow- up

5. Key worker policy

6. Patient information

7. Data collection, including procedures for confidentiality

8. Outline of other activities, e.g. teaching, training, CPD, audit and quality

9. Key meeting representation, e.g. Trust, network

10. Relationships with other key local service providers

Many teams in your locality will have operational policies and if in doubt, it may be worth asking to review some of these to inform your thinking when developing or updating your own.

Leadership and effective teams

Most senior clinicians in Palliative Care will take on some kind of leadership role. Good leadership is difficult and whilst a detailed exploration of leadership skills is beyond the scope of this book, it is useful to reflect on what makes leading a team or service difficult.

From the perspective of a medical consultant, the transition from specialist registrar to consultant can feel like a chasm and not dissimilar to that between medical student and junior doctor – you have the skills, but putting them into practice involves a huge learning curve. Other senior (non-medical) clinicians, without such formal training programmes (at the present time), may also experience a similar sense of transition as they start to take on more managerial roles, such as managing junior members of staff, particularly if they have not received training to adequately equip them to fulfil these roles. Effective senior management support is essential to support staff and ensure that they have or develop the skills that they require when taking on new and more senior roles.

Working closely as part of a multi-professional team, most team members will want to be liked and to get on with their colleagues. Whilst for the majority of the time this is feasible, there can be conflict with a leadership role, where at times the clinical lead may be required to make decisions that may not be popular or welcomed by other team members. Being an effective leader can at times feel difficult and very uncomfortable – it is useful to learn that this is inevitable and does not mean that you are not doing a good job.

Effective leadership requires you to understand the context in which you are working and the limits of your team and/or organization. To be a successful leader it is worth investing time in getting to know your team, your service, and your organization (or hospital Trust) – you need to understand your service and how it fits organizationally into your Trust. Hospital Trusts are large, complex organisations; unless you get some idea of how things work and fit together and of key dynamics and people, your ability to lead and develop your service will be more limited.

Frank Blackler, Professor of Organisational Behaviour at Lancaster University, has suggested that adaptive leadership is crucial. Factors that underpin adaptive leadership include:

1. Collaboration ('distributed leadership') – a process of facilitating shared priorities on a background of established routines or history. This process can be complex: participants may not know how to make good use of each others' distinct contributions; and collaborative projects typically encounter setbacks and frustrations, so it can be difficult to maintain enthusiasm for them.

2. Co-operation – a process where contributions are combined with a focus on a shared task.

3. Co-orientation or collaboration – a process where understandings are developed and contributions are re-considered in a broader context so that they are re-fashioned.

In the real world, people are all different and will have various approaches to a problem or issue and may never entirely agree. The process of co-orientation through dialogue enables people to relate to the problem, to explore how a system is working, and to develop a shared terminology in order to feel safe in identifying solutions to a problem.

However, leadership brings with it its own tensions; an effective leadership requires an ongoing complex balance or juggling, for example:

1. Knowing and being uncertainty

2. Shaping the new whilst working with reality

3. Enabling close working relationships with colleagues whilst maintaining a distance

4. Being a good employee whilst having time to yourself

At different times, you will find such tensions wearing and dispiriting – try not to be too hard on yourself and to seek support from outside of your team or organization in order to keep sane. The worst thing to do is to escape by 'being busy', working long hours, and losing all perspective!

Many people are conservative and resistant to change; this may manifest as feelings of loss in colleagues. Act on the insight that loss is the heart of resistance to change. It is crucial when developing your service to identify and acknowledge this change and also to concentrate on developing colleagues' leadership skills so such effects are minimised.

Effective teams

Effective leadership is a key component of effective teams. Effective teams have:

1. A valued purpose: individual and collective difference is worked through the life of the team
2. Agreed and measurable goals
3. Quick, clear, effective feedback
4. Cohesion and a sense of enjoyment
5. Respect and recognition

As a leader, you will be instrumental and crucial to developing the context in order for teams to function effectively. This requires an effective facilitation and an active followership – so get people on your side and don't try to go it alone. It may be helpful to explore whether your organization offers any management or leadership development programmes so that you can be supported to develop your skills.

Team members in difficulty

Regular supervision meetings can give an early warning for team members who are experiencing difficulties. In our experience, such situations are few and there is no evidence that palliative care staff are more or less stressed or prone to burn out than other health care professionals. One marker of staff who are in difficulty may be an increase in sick leave, and many acute NHS Trusts now have trigger systems in place to identify staff who have had over the 'expected' amount of sick leave; such triggers usually prompt a meeting to discuss the case and a discussion between the staff member and their line manager to try to identify issues or concerns. Other manifestations may be irritability, overconscientiousness, criticism of other team members, irregularity in time-keeping, as well as the more obvious tearfulness and loss of 'joie de vivre.'

One department which is frequently overlooked when staff members are in difficulty is occupational health (OH). Staff members have direct access to this department and are able to talk about work-related issues within a confidential framework. Such contacts are confidential, so unless the team member gives permission, OH staff are unable to inform managers that a member of staff has approached them for support. Access to counselling is often available through this route. A manager can refer a staff member in difficulty to occupational health and then the conversation is open. When you are a manager, it is possible to feel that a staff member who does not have insight into their difficulties can understate the impact of their reaction to stress on other team members to their GP or occupational health. If the stressed staff member is upsetting or undermining team cohesion, HR will often need to be involved. Some more enlightened departments will also provide access to complementary therapies that staff may utilize for relaxation – but in practice such opportunities are often limited.

Supervision and reflective practice

Supervision is used in counselling, psychotherapy, and other mental health disciplines, as well as in many other professions engaged in working with people who are distressed, troubled, or ill. The practitioner who is being 'supervised' meets regularly with another professional, not necessarily more senior, but normally with trained in the skills of supervision to discuss case-work and other professional issues in a structured way. This is often known as clinical or counselling supervision or consultation. The purpose is to assist the practitioner to learn from his or her experience and progress in expertise, as well as to ensure good service to the client or patient.

Clinical supervision has been recognized by nursing professional bodies (the Nursing and Midwifery Council and the Royal College of Nursing) as a supportive way to facilitate learning from experience. Although this can be undertaken as a multi-disciplinary exercise, it is most effective when limited to uni-professional settings, as the understanding of roles is a helpful part of the process.[1]

The importance of reflecting on what you are doing, as part of the learning process, has developed from the work of David Schön, who suggested that the capacity to reflect on action so as to engage in a process of continuous learning was one of the defining characteristics of professional practice[2]. *Reflective practice* is the ability to reflect *in* action (while doing something) and on action (after you have done it). It has become an important feature of professional

---

[1] http://www.wipp.nhs.uk/tools_gpn/toolu6_clinical_supervision_how_why.php
[2] Schön D A (1983) *The Reflective Practitioner: How Professionals Think in Action.* London: Temple Smith.

training programmes in many disciplines, and its encouragement is seen as a particularly important aspect of the role of the mentor of the beginning professional. It can be argued that 'real' reflective practice needs another person as mentor or professional supervisor, who can ask appropriate questions to ensure that the reflection goes somewhere, and does not get bogged down in self-justification, self-indulgence, or self-pity![3]

Ideally, palliative care team members should have access to clinical supervision or facilitated reflective practice to support their clinical (and other) roles, not only for talking through difficult scenarios, but also by having an independent person who is able to listen and facilitate the working through of an issue or problem. This section deals with clinical supervision and reflective practice from the context of a healthy team; more personal or individual issues are dealt with in Chapter 10.

Supervision is *not* about receiving advice or finding solutions to problems. Rather it should be seen as an opportunity to clarify thought processes and for the practitioner to decide on an appropriate solution. It is a multi-dimensional process which should provide the following:

1. An opportunity to review performance.
2. An opportunity to monitor levels and priorities of workload.
3. An opportunity to discuss individual cases.
4. The whole process should be supportive and educational, encourage motivation and enable a proactive approach to work.

The choice of supervisor is a critical one. The practitioner should have a supervisor he/she is comfortable with and one with whom they can develop a rapport. Equally the supervisor should have an understanding of the role of the supervisee. There is little to be gained from trying to tease out difficulties in practice if the supervisor has no understanding of the specialty. As with a counselling situation, there should be a form of contract between the two parties. The role and responsibilities of the supervisor should be set out. Equally they should not be asked to take on the role unprepared. Adequate training should be completed prior to taking on the role. It is a personal decision who a practitioner approaches to be their supervisor.

In practice the model of clinical supervision can be undertaken in different ways. It can be organised to give peer support either on a one-to-one basis or within the setting of a small group. Alternatively team supervision can be undertaken where the focus would be on the objectives of the team, rather than on one individual, or on discussing complex or challenging cases.

---

[3] *http://www.learningandteaching.info/learning/reflecti.htm*

Shadowing supervision is helpful where there are new team members, who work with an experienced nurse in order to understand the complexities of the role – a form of role modelling. This usually takes place during the induction period, but may continue for some time for more inexperienced team members.

No matter what type of supervision is undertaken, it should be evaluated on a regular basis to ensure it fulfils the aims and objectives of the process. It is of paramount importance that there is trust and mutual respect on all sides. The process should cover four key areas:

1. Clinical work

2. Professional standards

3. Personal growth and development

4. Evaluation of work performance

Effective participation in clinical supervision is seen as individuals demonstrating their accountability and taking responsibility for the continuous improvement of their practice.

There is more discussion of mentoring and clinical supervision in Chapter 10.

Appointing new team members

The success of a palliative care team depends on the skills, personalities and cohesion of its members. Unlike surgery (where skills with a knife), or oncology (where excellent technical skills), can partly compensate for poor communication and people management skills, there is no room for deficiencies in these areas in palliative care services. Team members need to be highly skilled professionals who can work as part of a team and be exemplary communicators. Within the environment of an acute hospital there may be some colleagues who are concerned about plans to develop palliative care services that may 'rob them of the control over patients'. There may be perceived threats to the autonomous care of their patients; equally there may be fears that the development of a new service or expansion of an existing service may call into question their skills and expertise or use up money that would otherwise finance their services. Good communication will be the best possible way to overcome these barriers.

If starting a new service where none has previously existed, decisions need to be made about the composition of the team, but should follow the framework outlined in the 2004 'Improving Outcomes Guidance', as discussed earlier. It is likely that in future any 'tariff' to fund for palliative care will be based on consultant episodes of care, but it is not yet clear whether this relates only to medical consultants. Consideration must also be given to the fact that once a team is established, the workload will invariably grow and where possible this should be factored in. In developing established services, you need first to consider your strategic aims and match the competencies of your existing team onto these, then consider what further staff you require to achieve your next steps. A further important influence on your plans will be the availability and type of accommodation for the team, such as where are any new staff members to be housed, in addition to 'on and set-up' costs, such as desks, chairs, computers, and printers to enable team members to work effectively. A PA, secretary, or administrator cannot work without a desk, computer, and 'phone. A specialist nurse may be able to share one for a short time, but it will not be satisfactory long-term arrangement. If the office is too noisy and crowded, difficult and sensitive phone conversations will be limited and confidentiality can be breached. Palliative care teams are resource expensive (e.g. staff) but only has its offices to work in; equipment and drugs are not significant parts of the therapeutic armamentarium in palliative care but skilled clinicians are.

A hospital palliative care service needs to be fully staffed with senior clinicians, in all disciplines, before it can employ those disciplines in training grades. Much of the time team members need to work alone seeing patients, and clinicians in other teams will not be able to 'check' their work, so a miscalculation in opioid conversion or an incorrect prescription for a syringe driver will not usually be picked up until another specialist sees their work the next day. It is not really helpful for first or even second year specialist registrars to work in the acute Trust as they will often not be confident enough of their decisions, medical or in difficult psychosocial situations, to enjoy it or for the team to feel entirely at ease.

Making appointments

Whoever is being appointed, it is essential to follow Trust policies on Recruitment and Selection, including Equal Opportunities legislation. For any new post, it is necessary to prepare a thorough job description and person specification; it can be useful to ask colleagues for example job descriptions, from previous successful appointments to use as a guide and a prompt for discussions as to the skill mix you are looking to recruit. There are also many sample job descriptions available through vacancy bulletins (e.g. *www. nhsjobs.net*) that can be scrutinized and adapted to suit your service. From a nursing and AHP perspective the job description and person specification will need to comply with the appropriate level on the Knowledge and Skills Framework (KSF) outline, and also fit the banding for Agenda for Change (AfC). For non-medical appointments, job descriptions then need to be sent to Trust Agenda for Change Banding committees for confirmation of the banding. Consideration should also be given, if you are considering extended team member appointments, e.g. social work and psychology, as to how these posts will integrate within the team and how they can be supported professionally within the organization.

You will also need to confirm funding arrangements with finance; will need to advertise following Trust guidelines (which may be costly and for some posts may need to come out of your budget); and will need to format your job descriptions according to Trust guidance.

Before advertising any post it is wise to seek advice from recruitment/HR, especially if it is not a mainstream post such as a CNS (e.g. end- of- life facilitator funded by your team on a temporary contract). Employment law is increasingly complex and there may well be hidden problems which you will need to overcome before the appointment.

It is also worth considering people's requests for flexible working and whether these can be accommodated within a team. If several part time appointments are being considered, then it is crucial to ensure that funding is available to ensure effective handover (if people are job-sharing) and that the service is adequately covered throughout the working week. Some services have creatively utilized volunteer therapists attached to the team who work on specific hours each week; by doing this it is possible to provide a comprehensive service but without too much initial financial burden. Further options include approaching departments, such as social work, to see if they would be willing to second a member of staff with the service on a given day.

If there are several part-time appointment and your team is small, remember to put the day on which the MDT is held as part of everyone's job plan so that there is one day when everyone is in. This will also help planning for team away days or team training, etc.

Once the job description has been drawn up, costed and banded, consideration should be given to the advertising process. Trust personnel departments will provide expertise in supporting the recruitment process and should be involved. Most Trusts now use online systems for applying for posts and the details will be included in the advert. Adverts should include the closing date and contact details of someone for people to contact for further information or for informal visits. When setting this up, make sure you have arranged the date when your entire panel can meet or you will find that the appointment committee may not be able to convene until some weeks/ months after the closing date; this is very unsatisfactory and you may lose excellent candidates to other jobs this way. In most NHS Trust non-medical posts are advertised internally as a given, but for any specialist appointments it is likely that national advertising, via the NHS jobs website *http://www.jobs.nhs.uk/* will also be required. For some specialist posts, such as social work or psychology, wider consideration should also be given to where to advertise, e.g. community care for social work staff.

Once the job description and advert have been written, and the job is ready to be advertised, make certain you can get requisite practitioners together to (i) shortlist and (ii) interview for the post in good time. It is very unsatisfactory for everyone if there is long gap between advertising and interviewing and may lead to you losing an outstanding candidate who accepts another post in this period.

It is essential that formal processes are followed for the appointment processes and any staff involved in the recruitment process should have received appropriate training (most NHS Trusts run recruitment and selection courses). The national guidance is that such training should be updated three-yearly. Prior to the closing date, you should consider who will be on the appointment panel; these panel members are involved in both the shortlisting and interview process. When shortlisting, all candidates have their applications measured against the person specification; current good practice is for applications to be anonymized in line with equal opportunities guidance, but this is not always feasible. Consideration should also be given to the structure of the interview: the panel should agree the questions in advance and the same panel member should ask the same question to each candidate to ensure equity. Some panels use a scoring system and/or make notes against each candidate's response to questions. For nursing posts it is not unusual for the candidates to be asked to give a short presentation on a particular subject. For a new service it is often useful to request candidates to give their vision for the first year; not only will this type of presentation showcase presentation skills, but it gives an insight into how this candidate may fit into a newly constructed team.

All notes made during interviews will need to be returned to HR after the interview and will be referred to in case of subsequent disputes.

If you are chair of a panel, do ensure that you understand how to conduct an interview; talk to someone in HR if you predict problems and read the references before the interview (without sharing contents with other panel members in either entirety), so that any areas of concern can be discussed during the interview.

Medical appointments

There is a formal, statutory process for the appointment of consultants in Palliative Medicine. In the first instance, a job description needs to be developed (generic guidelines are available from the Royal College of Physicians

(RCP) at *http://www.rcplondon.ac.uk/professional/aac/aac_consult.htm* and approved by the employing Trust. For NHS Trusts, once Trust approval has been obtained, the job description should be sent to the RCP Regional Specialty Advisor for College approval. (Note that this is not required for appointments made by Foundation Trusts, but we would regard it as good practice that this guidance still to be followed.)

Once the job description has been agreed with the Regional Specialty Advisor (see *http://www.rcplondon.ac.uk/regions/Regional Specialty Adviser*), the post can be advertised and an Appointment Advisory Committee (AAC) set up. The NHS (Appointment of Consultants) Regulations 1996 (amended 2004) states that an external assessor from the relevant College or Faculty should be included in the core membership of an AAC. Medical Staffing Departments should write to the College at least 6 weeks before the AAC date requesting nominations enclosing a copy of the job description and Regional Advisers correspondence. A list of up to 10 nominations will be drawn up by the RCP; representatives are all senior consultants who are also Fellows of the College. Trusts are given a set of nominations most suitable for their particular AAC together with a form to return to the College confirming the name of the consultant who agrees to represent the College. College representatives are full members of an AAC and should be included in the shortlisting process. The College representative at the SAC ensures that the candidate has the necessary qualifications and experience to undertake the advertised post.

The NHS good practice guidance on the appointment of consultants is available from the Department of Health (see *http://www.dh.gov.uk/prod_consum_ dh/groups/dh_digitalassets/@dh/@en/documents/digitalasset/dh_4102750.pdf*). It is important to note that NHS Foundations Trusts do not have a statutory responsibility to follow this guidance, although they can choose to do so.

Guidance is also available on the Royal College Physicians website for setting up staff grade/associate specialist posts in Palliative Medicine (see *http://www. rcplondon.ac.uk/professional/aac/aac_associate.htm* and *http://www.rcplondon. ac.uk/professional/aac/aac_staffgrade.htm*).

The appointment of doctors in training is co-ordinated through Foundation Schools or Postgraduate Deaneries - (see Chapter 8 for more information).

Consultant job plans

Consultants' timetables are governed by job plans that outline the balance of activities on a weekly basis. The week is broken down into programmed activities (PAs), which are of 4 hours duration each. A full- time consultant job will usually comprise 10 PAs (i.e. 40 hours/week). Sample job plans for physicians are available on the Royal College Physicians website, but in general terms are broken down into activities relating directly to clinical care (DCC) and supporting professional activities (SPA). In a standard consultant job plan, the ratio of DCC to SPA is around 7.5–8 DCC to 2.5–2 SPA. However, this ratio may not be appropriate for Palliative Medicine consultants, where contributions to teaching, training, and service development may be proportionately higher than for other consultants and it is important that when developing job plans and job descriptions, the balance effectively reflects what is required of that consultant appointment and that the Trust is aware of this. We are conscious that many acute Trusts may not understand the role of Palliative Medicine Physicians, many of whom will be working to job plans that do not accurately reflect their day- to-day jobs but who are under enormous pressure to increase their DCC over SPA. In these situations there may be opportunities through yearly appraisal and job plan reviews for job plans to evolve more appropriately and it is to be hoped that in the future there may be support and guidance available through the Association Palliative Medicine. If your appraising consultant is not in Palliative Medicine (which happens often), you can ask for another consultant colleague in the specialty to be present and it is also useful to or prepare a careful record of what you do and why.

Further information regarding job planning is available on the British Medical Association website at *http://www.bma.org.uk/employmentandcontracts/working_arrangements/job_planning/index.jsp*

Induction and mandatory training for staff

For any new members of staff, some thought needs to be given to induction programmes. Most NHS Trusts will run generic induction programmes that will also cover some aspects of mandatory training – these can vary from one day to two weeks and are usually different for different staff groups. These induction programmes are usually organized by postgraduate education departments in conjunction with personnel and by professional groups (for medical and nursing staff at least).

In addition to Trust induction, departments will also be asked to set up local induction programmes for new members. Local induction will usually include meetings with key members of staff, mandatory training that was not covered in Trust induction and potentially a visit to other local palliative care units or community teams. The needs of new staff members in familiarising themselves with a new organization, teams, and working practices has to be balanced with service needs, but you should anticipate that a new team member is unlikely to be fully functioning for at least a month.

It may be worth deferring some 'orientation' meetings for a month or even longer, e.g. with the Chair of the Trust or Chief Executive or Chief Nurse, so that the newly appointment consultant or CNS has something particular to comment on or some aspect of strategy they want to discuss. Meetings set up simply to meet other people who can fall a bit flat if there is nothing specific to discuss. This is obviously not true for individuals with whom the new person is going to start working straight away.

Mandatory training requirements will vary between professional groups and within organizations but are likely to include most of the following: basic life support, infection control, consent, devices (e.g. syringe drivers), manual handling, fire and safety, safeguarding adults and children, and use of relevant databases and electronic patient records. Most of these training requirements will need to be repeated on a regular (e.g. yearly) basis, and you should ensure that you are aware of the mandatory training requirements for the staff that you manage and that compliance with these requirements are reviewed during the appraisal process.

Case study: Teams in action

Julie was appointed as sole practitioner to a medium-sized (600 beds) Acute Hospital Trust. She had previously worked within a similar environment but in a different region. Although she had not worked in the specialty before, she had undertaken many courses and was well qualified to take up the post. The hospital had never had a specialist palliative care team before. Following induction she was ready to receive referrals, but they were slow coming in as clinicians were unused to having palliative care available. Gradually referrals were received and the service demand grew over a period of 6 months. An audit of referrals at this time indicated that the service was not able to meet demand; therefore a bid was drawn up for a second team member. Following successful recruitment, the service continued to grow and then required secretarial support. A grade 2 A&C post was created which meant that the phone was manned by a person when the team members were out of the office, improving the service. This seemed to have a very positive effect and the number of referrals increased once again.

A crisis in the local community team then saw a team of three reduced to a single-handed practitioner, Kate. For additional support Kate decided to approach her manager and request that she was temporarily housed within the hospital with the neighbouring team. This process worked so well that when additional team members were recruited, the team stayed together. This had the advantage of direct face-to-face communication between the hospital and community teams on a regular basis, which was found to be extremely beneficial for patient care.

This cohesive team has gone from strength to strength and now consists of eight members, four for the PCT and 4 for the acute Trust. 2 Consultants in Palliative medicine have also been appointed over time and they are also sited with the now integrated team.

There is now a comprehensive educational programme to help generalists in hospital and community improve their skills and regular journal clubs and audits of practice.

Chapter 3

Organizing clinical care

The best service is one that is responsive to patient (and referrer) needs and this requires flexibility: the more usual pattern in other specialities of rigidly designated sessions for clinics and formal ward rounds will delay patients' access to care. However, this flexibility needs to be balanced with some constraints which also operate to maintain or improve the quality of patient care:

1. Available resources; most teams at the moment work 9 am to 5 pm, and Monday to Friday with advice/visiting from consultants (or other team members) on-call outside these times.

2. The need for team members to have a manageable workload, reasonably predictable working hours, time to hold an MDT, and necessary team fixtures together.

3. Time to run an out-patient service.

4. Time to run education sessions so that in the longer-term the quality of 'generalist' palliative care in the hospital is improved for the benefit of all patients, most of whom are not referred to the support team.

5. Time for strategic work to improve access to, and co-ordination of, all palliative care services.

6. Time for research to inform clinical practice.

If you are setting up or remodelling a hospital palliative care team, do take some time to look at how others operate across the world. Routes of access to care can also be tailored to individual patient groups but also for different clinical teams which will have varying levels of interest and expertise in palliative care.

Models of care: delivering palliative care in the acute setting

In the UK, the traditional model is for hospital palliative care teams to work with other health care staff to provide specialist palliative care to patients in hospital. In some areas there may be no hospital team and under these circumstances the community team may be called upon to fulfil a dual role and provide an 'in reach' service to patients in hospital. Equally, the hospital team may provide 'outreach' to patients in a community setting if there is no dedicated community team. The range of services provided may vary but could consist of:

1. Specialist patient care such as advanced symptom management or expertise for complex psychosocial issues
2. Advice, support and education for patients and carers
3. Consultancy and education of other health care professionals
4. Liaison with services outside the hospital

Hospital palliative care teams will vary in composition, and may have a variety of titles. For example, where services have received pump prime funding from charities such as Macmillan Cancer Support, a requirement of the funding will be for Macmillan to remain in the title. Other services may refer to themselves as hospital support or hospital palliative care teams – but in essence, all are likely to be fulfilling similar roles. Some teams may wish members to have an active role and work alongside other health care professionals for a specific episode of care. Others may work more on a consultancy basis, and give advice only. Others again, may have non-medical prescribers as part of the team, and these personnel may prescribe specific medications for patients under their care.

Box 3.1 Example model of care: Advisory hospital palliative care team

- The team works in an advisory capacity with no dedicated beds – so patients remain under the care of the referring consultant.
- Team members are allocated set wards within hospital.
- Referrals are received in office and allocated according to above.
- Wards are visited each day to deal with referrals.
- Other referrals may be collected on 'ad hoc' basis during ward visits
- Advice is given on symptom management and on complex psychosocial issues and annotated on patient system (either notes or electronic system).
- Key issues are communicated to the referring team and other relevant health and social care professionals verbally.
- Follow-up is made at the discretion of the team member dependent on patients' palliative care needs.

There are compelling reasons for delivering palliative care in an advisory capacity in an acute-care setting and alongside other disciplines. By doing this, it keeps palliative care in the 'mainstream' where the expertise offered by the specialist teams' form an integral part of the day-to-day care of patients. Equally the non-specialist staff can develop their palliative care skills.

In addition to hospital palliative care teams working in an advisory capacity, some acute hospitals also have dedicated palliative care units within the hospital environment where patients are under the direct care of a palliative medical consultant for the duration of their stay. If designated beds are appropriate, a centre of excellence and teaching can develop. The pros and cons of specialist palliative care beds are debated further in Chapter 4.

Box 3.2 Example model of care: Palliative care unit

- Patients are admitted directly to the unit under the care of a consultant in Palliative Medicine.
- This may involve direct admission from Primary Care, in which case arrangements must be made for direct admission to the unit and not through an A&E department.
- Alternatively patients may be transferred from other wards as beds become available.
- If patients are 'outlying' on general wards and awaiting transfer, the hospital support team should ensure regular review.
- Daily multi-disciplinary ward round to review care.
- Weekly MDT discussion of all new referrals and complex cases.

There are some distinct advantages of following the 'consultation'-type approach rather than have beds within a dedicated unit:

1. As the patients are scattered throughout the hospital, there is no need to run and equip a dedicated unit.
2. There are numerous opportunities to impart knowledge to other health care professionals and underpin palliative and end-of-life care as an integral part of everyday practice.
3. The consultation service can influence the care of patients not directly referred to them by the 'ripple effect'. Established teams may well find they spend a great deal of time advising on the care of patients on the ward

they have been called to, but not necessarily only on the patient they were referred.

Equally there are advantages of having a dedicated palliative care unit:

1. The unit can be seen as a centre of clinical expertise for palliative care within the acute hospital Trust.

2. The administration of medications can be more controlled and is usually more appropriate - thereby supportive advanced symptom management for those patients with the most complex needs.

3. Formal bedside teaching and role-modelling can be undertaken.

4. There is a cohort of patients on whom it may be easier to undertake research, as they are under the direct care of a palliative care consultant.

5. Allied health care professionals and other professional support can be delivered within the unit.

6. There are opportunities for training hospital staff by offering placements on the unit.

Any successful palliative care team should provide a service based on a thorough needs assessment, and it is imperative that no matter what model is undertaken, that it fits the needs of requirements and resources of the organization. Care delivery will need to be flexible and have the capacity to adapt according to changing hospital priorities. By working closely with other disciplines a culture of respect and trust can be developed, and this is often the catalyst for early and appropriate referrals.

Developing services

Once a team is established, do not feel that its patterns of work should never change: clinical care changes in specialities as medical advances take place. Remember the impact of anti-retrovirals on human immunodeficiency virus (HIV) care; consider the impact of rituximab and other biological therapies on the management of advanced non-Hodgkin's lymphoma (NHL) and other cancers.

Keep your pattern of work under review and ensure you are meeting patients, carers and referrers' needs. This can be done by:

1. *Satisfaction surveys:* Ideally these should be carried out, distributed, or collected by someone outside the team, e.g. Patient Advice and Liaison Services (PALS), but in practice this may not be possible. There are limitations to a team managing a satisfaction survey themselves, for example, patients will not usually be critical of the team caring for them. Ideas for how to run and manage satisfaction surveys can be found on the Macmillan Cancer Support (see *www.macmillan.org.uk*) or National Council for Hospice and Specialist

Palliative Care Services website (at *www.nchspcs.org.uk*). Honest feedback from patients and carers needs to be a cornerstone of service design. You can also involve 'users' (perhaps from the network groups) to scrutinise your ideas and help you improve communication with patients on improving services.

2. *Measuring your impact:* It is really important to know the sort of impact your care is making on the problems for which patients are referred to you. This is difficult as there is no perfect way of doing this: introducing lots of outcome measures can add significant time to consultations without giving useful data. Often the baseline measure is done but not the follow-up. None of us have solved this problem yet, but it is important that you try to assess it. Process audits can be important: one of us has found it useful to have it documented that 100% of patients with symptom control problems are seen within 24 hours of referral, 90% on the same day and the other 10% receiving immediate telephone advice. You need some sort of data that show that you are being responsive to clinical needs.

3. *Liaison with referrers:* If your colleagues do not feel they get the help they need but only what you choose to give them, your reputation will suffer and you will not be meeting part of the remit of a consultation service. The word service is important: if this is interpreted as 'slavish', you will end up with team members working very long hours, only seeing patients for extended periods until everything in their care is 'perfect' and the team will collapse. If the opposite holds and members try to contain their workload by telling everyone who refers that 'they do not fit our criteria' or 'we have a meeting and cannot come until next week' this will be equally damaging.

Find ways to make sure you are supporting your colleagues adequately in the care of their patients (many of whom you will not need to see). You could run surveys, ask to go to a team meeting to collect their views, run a half day where team representatives come to set out what they feel is done well and what else would help them. Think broadly and inventively about this: look at ways this sort of information is collected by other services (e.g. liaison psychiatry) and what is in the literature.

Documentation

As the majority of hospital palliative care teams work in an advisory capacity, there is a need for some documentation of activity that is separate from the patients' case notes. This may be using paper notes or an electronic record, or a mix of both. What should be documented and in what form is a complex issue, particularly if teams are working across organizations and there is a need to streamline documentation.

After the Climbié enquiry it was recommended that information in one specialty's notes should be available to everyone and that separate notes with separate information was not acceptable. This does cause concern for services like palliative care that have access to very sensitive information. Talk to the Caldicott Guardian at your Trust for advice on how to keep your notes legal and helpful for patient care.

Referral documentation

In many areas, services have worked collaboratively to develop shared referral criteria and documentation, e.g. referral pro formas. For example, all the specialist palliative care services in south London use the same referral form and work to the same referral criteria. The palliative care services in Kent have also developed shared referral criteria and a network proforma. For one of the authors, four services in her locality had separate referral forms. However, with co-operation from all teams, an integrated referral form was developed meeting the needs of all services across the locality. This has had the added benefit of being available electronically, so referrals can now be completed online and emailed to a central point for each service. Onward referrals, for example when an episode of care has been completed in hospital and patients are to be transferred to Primary Care, can be done quickly via the electronic system, although some staff may still like to security of having a paper copy of a referral. An example of a referral proforma is shown in Appendix 1.

Team documentation

Most hospital teams are consultative and will write in the patient case notes, but many also duplicate this by recording contact information in palliative care notes or databases. It can be important to have such a parallel system in order to support out of hours working and for quality and audit purposes, however it can mean that valuable clinical time is spent documenting contact information in different places. Some teams routinely fax copies of their documentation in the patient notes to their office to minimize this duplication, which works well for them, but results in large amounts of paper to manage.

There is no perfect system and individual teams need to work out:

1. The amount of clinical information needed in their own notes for continuity of care and joint working in the team.
2. What is needed for out of hours care.
3. What needs to be collected for national and local audits, including activity data. This sort of information needs to be easily retrievable from your records and preferably filled in contemporaneously.

Electronic records

More and more services are moving towards an integrated IT system, where all areas of service can access a single patient record, which is live and dynamic. Although none of the authors are working with fully integrated palliative care IT systems at the present time, they are being developed and piloted in many areas of the UK and abroad. The advantage of this is that the different parts of a palliative care service can view up-to-date interventions with patients. This has the potential to prevent duplication, ensure effective communication, and has the potential for audit and service evaluation. Comprehensive electronic records also enable remote access to support out of hours working, via the use of cryptocards or virtual private networks. The use of an electronic patient record/database is helpful for statistical analysis of services, such as the data collection required for the minimum data set returns for National Council for Hospices and Specialist Palliative Care (NCHSPC), thereby removing the onerous task of manual collection of data.

Most acute hospital Trusts now have electronic patient records (EPR) and increasingly, documentation during episodes of care are recorded electronically rather than in the patients' case notes. This poses challenges – for example, multidisciplinary team meeting (MDM) outcomes will need to be incorporated in to the EPR, but the opportunities for sharing of clinical information are manifest.

As with any IT system, particularly one holding sensitive patient data, safeguards must be in place to ensure the safety of the data. Caldicott guidelines must be adhered to. Equally, in the light of so many recent losses of sensitive data on portable devices, it is of paramount importance that all data is securely stored with password protection being a minimum standard. It should be recommended that before using any IT devices to store patient data the security measures are discussed with IT departments.

Most Trusts will not allow individuals to take named patient data offsite in a USB key (unless encrypted) and any notes needed for home visits will need to be kept in a locked bag at home or when carried in the car or other transport.

The referral process

It is generally quicker and more streamlined to have an electronic system for referrals. However, not all teams will have the capacity (or, in some instances, the capability) of developing an electronic system. In practice, any referral process needs to be flexible to best meet the needs of the organization and to minimize delays in responding to patients' needs.

Methods of referral may include

1. The EPR
2. Use of a referral bleep
3. Single fax or telephone number
4. Face to face (common in practice, though you can ask individuals to phone all the details to the office if you are in the middle of seeing someone else; this is a good way of getting background information that is not put on forms quickly)
5. Via a referral form

Some teams may allocate a team member to be the 'emergency contact' or to be responsible for triage of referrals for the day. However if referrals are made and details have to be passed on, it is important to ensure secure transfer of sensitive data.

Many teams ask for referrals to be made using a standardized pro forma or referral form to ensure that all necessary details are transferred to the team. This can be transmitted to the team electronically (via the hospital EPR) or by fax. However the standard of the referral will be very dependent on who is completing the form! Not all hospitals teams, however, use referral forms as they may be seen by staff as a relative barrier to referral and to potentially slow down the referral process.

In our experience, staff are increasingly used to using the EPR for referral to many services and this enables key information to be communicated; however, the team need to be alert to collecting these referrals from a central point to minimize delays.

Telephone referrals can also be phoned to a central point. With appropriate training a good team secretary can be on hand to take referrals rather than have an answer phone. One advantage of this is that she/he can ask for all pertinent information.

If the team has clerical/secretarial support, he/she should have some way of communicating urgent messages to team members; mobile phones are now standard equipment for all staff in the community and bleeps or pagers in the hospital setting. This is particularly important in the community for safety and is a requirement of most 'lone worker' policies.

Where referrals are able to be made by telephone, administrative support is vital. The advantages of administrative support include:

1. Patients, relatives, or clinical staff ringing into services are reassured by human contact.
2. The secretary taking the call can get hold of a clinician in an emergency.

3. Time is saved as giving clinical advice is separated from taking down necessary information; the secretary cannot get involved in clinical discussions.

4. The uncertainty of leaving a message on an answering machine is diminished.

There are important standards that need to be maintained if this system is to work.

1. The secretary needs to demonstrate both empathy and understanding. He/she needs a calm manner and good communication skills, as he/she will take calls from distressed relatives. Secretaries may therefore require support /coaching/ clinical supervision and should be offered the opportunity to debrief after difficult phone calls.

2. The referrer must give clear guidance on how urgent the referral is: it is unfair for the secretary to have to gauge this: a specific question must be used such as; 'Does the patient need seeing today?'

3. The secretary will generally be helped by having a 'script' or proforma or guidance on how to take down referrals so that no information is left out.

4. Locum or bank staff who are asked to fill this role temporarily need to have some training beforehand: for planned absences they should spend some time with the regular secretary before taking over in their absence.

When there is no administrative support, systems should be put into place for one team member to collect messages during the day.

This may be:

1. Via remote access to an answer phone

2. By physically returning to the office at set times during the day

Team answerphone messages must be clear that messages are picked up intermittently (preferably stating when) and giving a pager or mobile phone number as an alternative for urgent enquires. This phone will then need to be set to receive messages as it is not feasible to have constant interruptions in the working day to take phone calls from colleagues.

Referral criteria

It is important to have explicit referral criteria. Most palliative care networks have developed these criteria and wherever possible these criteria should be used to avoid confusion. Where you have major concerns about them, raise the issues with the network group for consideration in the first instance!

It may also be helpful to consider how you will categorize referrals (e.g. routine or urgent) and how you will respond to them.

The referral guidelines from Merseyside and Cheshire Palliative Care Network group are reproduced below.

Box 3.3 Example: Referral criteria

- For patients with advanced, progressive, incurable, malignant, and non-malignant disease who have complex physical, psychological, spiritual, social, or carer needs
- Where the patient and/or families needs cannot be met by health care professionals in the current care setting and may be met by a specialist palliative care service, is this a direct quote? Otherwise would suggest a change
- Where the current health care professionals require support and advice of the specialist palliative care service

Choice of service

The service to which the patient is referred may vary according to

- Individual patient acceptance of that service
- Available service development within the area
- Local integration of services

Ideally the patient would be referred to the integrated palliative care service who as a team would assess the patient needs and offer appropriate services to meet those needs.

Aim

- To provide specialist support working alongside health care professionals in primary care, hospital, or in other care setting

Admission to service

- Takes place at time of recognition of specialist palliative care needs by health care professionals

Discharge from service

- Takes place when patient, family, and associated health care professionals no longer require specialist palliative care input

Managing team workload day to day

The work of the team needs to be managed so that:

1. Patients' needs are assessed rapidly by an appropriate member of staff and seen as quickly as their condition dictates (e.g. the team may assess over phone that the patient should not be seen until they have had chance to discuss possible oncological treatment with the specialist if newly diagnosed and came in on take with what seemed innocuous symptoms).

2. Patients get good continuity of care, even if not seen by the same team members each time.

3. Team members can get non-clinical aspects of their work (which generally help longer-term aims of team) accomplished in a timely, unhurried way.

4. Team members are not put under undue stress and there is enough time in the week for the team to meet together to accomplish for clinical and non-clinical work priorities.

5. Team members give and receive mutual support.

Palliative care support team work is very variable, sometimes it is very busy and then it may be quiet. You may be staffed adequately but then a constellation of mischances occur together (illness plus compassionate leave plus unfilled post). Team members need to be able to adapt and re-prioritize work as needed. They may start a working day with a full diary and then a clearly urgent referral comes, which may take some time even if dealt with efficiently (e.g. young dying person who wants to get home ASAP after change of heart re treatment).

Communication and cohesion needs to be good enough for everyone to be able to say 'yes I can take on some of your patient load to enable you to see the urgent referral' or 'I cannot take on anyone else but perhaps I could ....'. Team members need to able to believe the person who says they can do no more as resentment will build up if one person is always doing the extra work.

It is difficult to build and to maintain such a team spirit; don't be disheartened if things are not working that way but continue to examine practice and work on ways to achieve this spirit. Good team structures can contribute to this feeling of fairness and meetings can be part of this. However, if you have too many meetings, people cannot get on with their work and referrers will feel palliative care is unavailable. If you have too few, the team will become atomised and in time demoralised and there will not be the support when there are difficult times or patients with very difficult problems.

Clinical team meetings

The following are suggested as the sorts of meetings you will need to run efficiently and meet NICE guidance. Do be circumspect about the number of regular meetings (you will find that you need ad hoc ones anyway): the authors mostly favour minimizing the number of fixed points in the week because of the variability of support team work (see later).

1. *Morning briefing:* For those working clinically or senior supervising physician/nurse.
   i. Review current caseload.
   ii. Discuss new referrals.
   iii. Allocate/prioritize the day's work.
   iv. Diary meeting for non-clinical work/other commitments.

   Length 1/2 to 1 hour maximum

2. *Possible lunch-time briefing:* Some teams may wish to catch up quickly in the middle of the day, to assess progress and re-prioritize when necessary.

   Length 1/2 hour maximum

3. *Multi-disciplinary team (MDT) meeting (see later):* One weekly; main clinical team meeting of the week.

4. *Multi-professional review:* Team ward rounds/joint visits; weekly or as needed. Some teams will organize ward rounds with the senior doctor and nurses seeing patients with complex needs: this allows multi-professional review.

Other teams may organize 'joint visits' as and when needed. It is important to make sure that 'joint visits' do occur; it gives the opportunity for team members to work with and learn from each other. Without this, team members can become 'lone workers' and in time they may become 'fossilized', using the same techniques and failing to progress and develop.

Ward rounds/meeting with other teams

The authors work in services where they undertake joint ward rounds on the oncology ward or attend other teams' ward meetings. These rounds can be important in building relationships and in communication, especially if you are invited to joint meetings where there are a high proportion of patients needing palliative care. However, it is very easy for the team to spend too much time attending team meetings (to tick a box on NICE guidance form) when they cannot contribute much or their contribution can be offered in another way (e.g. rapid access to outpatients). This happens when:

1. Patients do not have active palliative care problems but may need referral in the future.

2. Patients are merely referred for palliative care but there is no discussion of their problems.
3. Only one or two patients have palliative care problems in an hour's meeting.

You may wish to suggest that instead of attending the MDT or ward round that

1. Any patients with immediate palliative care needs can have rapid access to a palliative care out-patient clinic.
2. Palliative care patients are discussed at the beginning of the MDT so that team member can use time efficiently, leaving after they are discussed.
3. Advice is given on a prn basis, for example, many patients discussed at the upper GI MDT are 'not fit for surgery' and are therefore designated 'for palliative care' but they do not necessarily have active palliative care needs and the important communication is between the MDT and the GP.

Review meetings regularly: what is a good use of time in 1 year may not be effective 2 years later. Clinical practice may have changed, you may have greater or fewer numbers of team members or different team members. Make sure that team members feel work is allocated fairly otherwise resentment will build up, possibly subliminally leading to team splits and discord.

Key workers

You will probably want to run a 'key worker' system with certain team members (clinical nurse specialists or specialist registrars) holding 'case loads' and others working as 'consultants' particularly those who have a significant proportion of strategic work

Patients may be allocated as they are referred or it is often useful for individual nurse specialists to cover designated wards or clinical areas. The nurse specialist can rotate round these designated areas so that no one feels that they 'own' certain wards or specialities and to prevent wards only wanting one particular nurse seeing their patients.

The NICE Improving Outcomes Guidance on Supportive and Palliative Care recommends that palliative care services are provided to enable 7 day per week visiting with 24-hour access to advice. Meeting these standards are challenging for most hospital palliative care services and are likely to require that services in a locality work collaboratively: most cancer and palliative care networks have teams addressing these issues in their area. An example of one model which meets the guidance is described in the next example. In pooling resources to cover weekends and bank holidays, it is of paramount importance that there are sufficient numbers of clinicians in each team to meet normal requirements and maintain team cohesion as well.

Box 3.4 Example: Delivering 7-day a week visiting and 24-hour telephone advice

Across two acute hospital Trusts (with three hospital sites), the four specialist registrars provide a visiting service to hospital patients with specialist palliative care needs at weekends between 9 am and 5 pm. Patients are highlighted for review by the hospital palliative care teams on the Friday afternoon and all relevant information is faxed to the on call registrar. The on call registrar is contactable via mobile phone and it is highlighted that they are required to travel between sites so may not be able to visit immediately to respond to an urgent call. The registrar is supported by a consultant on call. In addition to reviewing patients highlighted by the hospital teams, the registrars do also give advice and assess new referrals if they are prioritized as urgent. The on call registrar completes an on call record form for all patient contacts, which is faxed to the hospital teams, supported by a telephone handover on the Monday morning.

Seven days a week, consultants across three acute hospital Trusts (four hospital sites and three community palliative care teams) participate in an on call rota, providing 24-hour telephone advice to healthcare professionals for patients known to the hospital or community palliative care teams. All contacts are recorded on an on call record form and faxed to the relevant team the following morning, supported by telephone feedback if required.

This model of collaborative working across services enables us to meet the Improving Outcomes Guidance and supports the management of complex patients.

The multi-disciplinary team meeting

In the UK, the Palliative Care Service standards (developed from the NICE Improving Outcomes Guidance) require the palliative care multi-disciplinary team (MDT) to hold a weekly MDM, with both core and extended members present and attendance registered. Core members are required to attend at least 50% of meetings. Attendance is also required from a palliative care practitioner at some cancer-specific MDT meetings (see Chapter 4). This obviously will place additional burden on teams, but is valuable as patients who may require a palliative care intervention can be identified early. Monitor how the clinician's expertise is used at individual tumour site MDTs (see above) and provide input another way if necessary.

The palliative care MDM needs administrative support in order to function effectively. This task may fall to a dedicated MDT coordinator or may in some instances be taken over by the team secretary. It is common place for specific patients to be discussed at MDT. An example of who should be discussed can be seen below.

Box 3.5 Example: Kind of patients/carers being deiscussed

Patients/carers are discussed at the MDT as follows:

- All newly referred patients after initial assessment
- Patients with difficult symptoms or complex needs
- Patients whose family members or carers have complex needs, including high bereavement risk
- Patients being discharged/transferred (or have died)
- Patients going across care boundaries
- Other patients and families/carers as determined locally

The MDM discussion needs to include the spectrum of palliative care interventions and an action plan developed. In practice, most services use a proforma to support this, with key headings including:

1. Physical symptoms
2. Psychological issues
3. Social issues
4. Information needs
5. Spiritual issues
6. Carer concerns

The MDM action plans/outcomes need to be recorded in the patients' case notes or EPR, so that all teams involved in the patients' care are aware of the palliative care involvement and plans. One of us achieves this by printing the completed proforma (including the action plan) on yellow paper, which is then filed in the patients' notes by the team member undertaking the next assessment; the use of coloured paper ensures that the outcomes are clearly visible.

The MDM can be time- and labour-intensive; in one of our services with approximately 100 referrals a month and an average caseload of 30 to 40 patients, we now have two MDMs: one to discuss all patients on the caseload (this meeting can take several hours) and a further MDM to discuss all deaths and discharges. Despite this time involved, the MDM process is incredibly valuable by ensuring comprehensive MDT discussion, involvement of all team members, and a focus on key issues. It also provides a forum for reflection and support for team members, particularly for more complex cases. An example MDM proforma is shown in Appendix 2.

Discharging patients

Patients may be discharged from hospital palliative care services when they leave hospital, die, or are identified as having no ongoing specialist palliative care needs. In the last case, it is important to clearly communicate with the referring team so that they are aware of why the patient has been discharged.

Communicating with other services

When patients are discharged from hospital, adequate communication with other teams is essential and processes need to be put in place to achieve this communication. Where patients are being referred on to other palliative care services, e.g. hospice or community teams, a referral form will usually need to be completed and faxed or sent electronically to the relevant service. In our experience, it is also useful to send further supporting information, such as the hospital discharge notification letter (this usually includes the drugs on discharge), results of recent investigations, and relevant clinic letters/MDM outcomes. Hospital discharge letters or notifications rarely contain any detail of palliative care interventions during an admission; information that may be very useful for palliative care services and that may reduce duplication. We have therefore found it useful to send a palliative care discharge letter to the GP, hospice, or community palliative care team using a standardised proforma with the same headings as outlined in the section on the palliative care MDM. This is usually dictated by the key worker, but in more complex cases more than one team member contribute to the letter. This level of communication requires adequate administrative support so that it does not become unnecessarily burdensome for team members. Feedback from primary care and community palliative care teams, however, suggests that distinct palliative care communication is helpful and valued. In line with NHS policy, patients should be asked if they would wish to receive a copy of this correspondence.

In practice many patients move between settings and will be known to other palliative care services. Early notification from community palliative care teams that patients have been admitted and identification of key, pertinent issues can help continuity of care; some community services use admission notification pro formas, which we have found very useful and save multiple phone calls to chase up-to-date information. Once these patients are discharged back to the community services, effective communication to the community teams is also essential – we have found that palliative care discharge letters as described above can support this.

Bereavement services

Providing bereavement follow-up is challenging for hospital palliative care teams but should be considered. As a starting point, it is helpful to understand how the bereavement services in your organisation work and to explore whether other specialist services, e.g. paediatrics, cancer, have additional processes in place. The Trust bereavement office and chaplaincy team are a good place to start to collect this information.

Hospital palliative care teams may want to consider what level of bereavement support or follow-up they want and can provide. Examples include:

1. Involving an assessment of bereavement risk in the MDM discussion

2. Sending a standard bereavement letter to bereaved family members or informal carers to acknowledge their loss and offer generic information regarding bereavement

3. Inviting families and carers to bereavement meetings

4. Proactively following up family members/carers by telephone contact or visits

5. Organizing memorial services

6. Sending anniversary cards at 1 year

All of these interventions require staff training, systems to be put in place to support them and adequate administrative support. In some services bereavement follow-up is co-ordinated by palliative care social workers, but not all hospital teams have social work support and this may limit the follow-up that can be provided. It is also important to balance the time required to provide any form of bereavement follow-up with the demands of the day to day workload – in our experience, it can be difficult to prioritize bereavement calls when there are urgent issues arising across the hospital.

Summary

Clinical work needs to be organized to fit the needs of the patients that you see and in tune with the culture of your Trust. It also needs to be structured so that 'meetings' do not get in the way of a rapid, flexible clinical response: the organization of clinical care will need review to make sure that changes inside or outside the palliative care team have not made the current processes obsolete.

Chapter 4

Being part of the mainstream in the acute hospital

Being part of the mainstream in an acute hospital is essential for the survival and effective functioning of a hospital palliative care team. However, the nature of most hospital palliative care, where the clinicians are working in a predominantly advisory role, poses specific challenges. In the UK, few hospital palliative care teams have access to specialist palliative care beds; this is much more the norm in North America and across Europe. In UK hospitals, where organizational culture and targets are driven by bed-derived income and hospital statistics are derived from consultant admissions and outpatient visits, it can be easy for a hospital palliative care team, working in a purely advisory capacity, to struggle to figure on the hospital's radar. The issue of whether having beds in a dedicated unit, or as part of another clinical area, and how this impacts on 'being part of the mainstream' will be discussed later in this chapter.

However, all the authors are members of thriving, successful hospital palliative care teams that are well integrated into their respective hospitals. What are the keys to such success?

Key elements for successful integration can be seen as:

1. The public face of the team
2. Maintaining a high profile
3. Taking all opportunities for service development

The public face of the team

Flexibility, approachability, profile, and responsiveness are essential for successful integration. People need to know who you are, how to get hold of you and be confident that you can respond quickly, particularly in a crisis.

In our services, ways of raising and maintaining profile that we have found helpful include:

1. A laminated 'How to Access' card, printed on bright yellow paper, is displayed on wards and in other key clinical areas. These clearly need to be up to date and visible, as they can get buried under other information on ward notice boards.

2. A folder on the Trust intranet, available to all Trust staff, containing all key and relevant documentation.

3. Easy referral pathway – whilst some services insist on completion of a paper or electronic referral form, these can also be perceived as a barrier to referral. Individual services have to balance the desire for clear, appropriate referrals containing pertinent information with highly flexible access, with the downside that the result may be a relative paucity of information or poor quality of referral. Over the years the methods by which people can refer have increased (currently via pager, bleep, telephone call, fax, in person or via the electronic patient record), which may result in confusion. As a result of this, one of us has recently been piloting a referral triage system – see case study 'Referral Triage Pilot' for more details.

4. Clinical nurse specialists carry caseloads on designated wards, thereby enabling them to build lasting working relationships with ward staff. Being high profile in clinical areas, undertaking thorough clinical assessments, and teaching, all appear to lower the threshold for referral to palliative care and reduce the number of 'they're not ready for you yet' concerns. Rotation of individuals may be necessary if a culture starts developing where the ward is only pleased to see that one nurse, e.g. 'X looks after our patients.'

5. Take opportunities to advertise your service – in one of our Trusts we had a stand at the main entrance to coincide with World Hospice and Palliative Care Day (see case study 'World Hospice and Palliative Care Day').

Case study: Referral triage pilot

The triage concept uses a single 'triage' bleep, held on rotation by team members, whose responsibility is to receive and triage referrals. The person on triage needs to be available to take and see urgent referrals and attend team 'handover' meetings, in the morning and at lunchtime, to be aware of the workload of team members. The triage bleep holder, on receipt of a referral may:

1. give telephone advice,

2. undertake an initial assessment to assess whether the referral is appropriate,

3. pass non-urgent referrals to the team member best placed to respond, and

4. respond, as soon as possible, to an urgent referral, including in outpatients or the Emergency Department

In initial piloting, one of the problems encountered has been variable responses to the triage process from different team members, which has not been popular with all members of the hospital palliative care team. However, it has been very well received by clinical colleagues, several of whom have been extremely impressed by the speed of response to referrals, particularly in outpatient clinics. One concern, expressed by team members has been that the triage process, rather than streamlining as intended, introduced an extra layer of process, which was unhelpful.

Case study: World Hospice and Palliative Care Day

Each year, October sees World Hospice and Palliative Care Day (*http://www.worldday.org/*). This is an opportunity for your team to re-launch or advertise to a wide audience the services that you offer. In one of our Trusts, in 2008, we had a stand in the main entrance, close to the outpatient department, with relevant posters, leaflets, DVDs, and other literature available. Team members manned the stand, supported by the Chaplaincy team, members of our linked academic department and staff from a local end of life care modernisation programme. The stand was visited by patients, caregivers, and staff members, many of whom were asking basic questions about what palliative care is and the services on offer. Following on from this day, teaching requests have been received from staff groups that will help to inform the team's teaching programme over the coming year.

Maintaining a high profile

In order to become known, the hospital palliative care team needs to be visible and seen around the Trust. This can be achieved in a number of ways:

Cancer multidisciplinary meetings

When starting out it seems sensible to target cancer multidisciplinary meetings (MDMs) where the majority of appropriate referrals will be received, which are those of the common cancer types such as lung, breast, GI, and urology. It is also an effective use of time to focus on MDMs that are relevant for the patient profile of a hospital – so in one of our organizations, one of us spends several hours a week attending hepato-pancreato-biliary (HPB) MDMs, as the Trust is the network centre for HPB oncology.

In our experience, this time is well-spent for profile and for promoting Palliative Medicine as a specialty, but the number of referrals per meeting may be small, which makes it labour-intensive. It may help for a relatively senior clinician to attend these meetings to build links and maintain a high-profile, but cancer MDMs are also good opportunities for teaching and training for more junior staff. One author's department now goes only to selected meetings.

Targeting key clinics or ward rounds

One way to integrate into the mainstream is by developing outpatient palliative care clinics alongside existing clinics, such as oncology and regional neurology clinics. This has enabled us to run outpatient services and receive a steady stream of referrals by attendance in the same clinic area as other clinicians. In one of our services, involvement in the regional MND clinic has developed to the extent that assessment by Palliative Care is included in the multi-professional documentation and is mandatory for all patients with predominantly bulbar disease having assessments for enteral feeding or non-invasive ventilation.

One of us has also successfully built links with our regional haemato-oncology service by attending the weekly haemato-oncology ward round. This has led us to provide an acute symptom control service to the haemato-oncology patients, including those undergoing bone marrow transplantation (see case study in Chapter 1).

Management meetings and responsibilities

Organizational structures within hospitals will vary, but it is crucial that the structure relevant for the Palliative Care Team in your organization is defined and that you attend key management meetings. This enables dialogue with managers and clinicians, helps maintain a high profile and gets Palliative Care onto people's agendas. Relevant meetings may include hospital cancer committees and management meetings within the hospital management structure.

We have also found it useful to target meetings to undertake presentations around key areas, such as the results of the recent national Liverpool Care of the Dying Hospital audit. This enables a dialogue and sharing of ideas to get buy-in to strategic priorities.

As you become more established as a senior clinician in a hospital palliative care team, opportunities will also arise to take on more managerial roles and responsibilities within your organization. Whilst these opportunities may be time-consuming and not be to everyone's taste or skills, it can be a way of increasing your profile (and thereby that of the team) and promoting your specialty. We are aware of several hospital palliative care consultants that have risen through the ranks of hospital management to become clinical and subsequently medical directors of their organizations; such a profile can only be positive for the services they represent.

Presentation at key events

Medical consultants, as a member of the consultant body in a hospital, will find themselves on the rota for presentation at hospital grand (or staff) rounds. Attendance at these is also useful, not only in terms of continuing professional development (CPD) but also for networking with colleagues. We found presentations at these meetings to be a very useful forum for raising issues to the wider medical body, such as the implications of the Mental Capacity Act.

Demonstrate what you do

It is important to be able to demonstrate what you do, especially in a world now focussed on income generation and targets. The development or purchase of a database enables recording of all clinical activity, with the potential to produce annual reports, participation in National Council for Palliative Care Minimum Dataset returns and also enables regular monitoring of referral trends.

One of us sends our annual reports to a range of senior clinicians within our organization, in addition to other local services and the cancer network; we are surprised at how many letters and emails we have received over the years commenting on the content of the report – it certainly seems to be a useful tool to maintain profile.

In one of our organizations, with support from the Business Development Unit, we have been able to use our database to capture performance information that feeds into the monthly performance monitoring which is required by the Trust. We are now using the database to record contacts on the Private Patients ward, in order to be able to charge for this activity.

Most hospital support teams now use databases, either purchased or developed internally. Operating a predominantly paper system, as some services still do, means that the opportunities for detailed performance review and for clearly demonstrating clinical activity are reduced.

Hospitals will continue to be major providers for Palliative Care for the foreseeable future. Therefore the provision of high quality end of life and palliative care will be a priority for all Trusts. Providers should ensure that discussion and review of their service is undertaken at Board level at least annually.[3]

Engagement with those in training

Whilst it may seem to be a time-consuming exercise in a busy day, it is often useful for a member of the palliative care team to have a presence at the induction programme for new staff. Not only does this give an opportunity for a brief introduction to the service, but it enables new starters to put a face to a name of at least one team member.

Likewise having regular input into nurse and medical student training encourages the philosophy of palliative care to be embedded before preconceptions have a chance to become entrenched.

Taking all opportunities for service development

You need to try to identify and respond positively to opportunities for service development. These are a great way of linking with existing services and working strategically, although enthusiasm must be tempered with a degree of realism about what can be achieved within existing resources. However, service developments may also provide an opportunity to successfully argue for resources to support them.

With the increase in knowledge regarding the palliative care needs of non-cancer patients and the inclusion of palliative care in several UK national service frameworks (e.g. cardiac, COPD, renal, long-term conditions), there are opportunities to liaise with colleagues in other specialties to increase the availability to specialist palliative care. Further opportunities have arisen since the publication of the UK National End of Life Care strategy in 2008.[1]

Case study: Service development in practice

In one of our organisations, we were able to capitalise on the expansion and remodelling of an existing renal low clearance clinic to provide specialist input to the clinic and train a renal low clearance nurse specialist in palliative care; these developments have been mirrored as part of a funded modernisation initiative at a neighbouring acute hospital Trust. This initiative was successful as it came with an enthusiasm and will to work collaboratively from the renal team, whilst in palliative care we were able to find a team member (a SpR) who was keen to take on a new challenge. The outcome has been several years of successful joint working, which has evolved and the SpR involved in setting it up has now completed a PhD on renal palliative care.

Beds or no beds

Most hospital palliative care services in the UK operate in an advisory capacity as hospital support teams. However, some hospitals have had specialist palliative care beds for many years (such as the Royal Marsden in Chelsea and Sutton), and some have more recently opened dedicated palliative care units (e.g. the Macmillan Unit at the Northern General in Sheffield) and others dedicated beds in oncology wards (e.g. at Basildon, Guy's, and Bristol hospitals).

There is clearly a strong argument for working in an advisory capacity, allowing the palliative care resources to spread across an organization, thereby working through information exchange, partnership and education to increase the generalist skills of hospital staff. For the majority of patients, this way of working is effective but there might be some patients, with complex specialist palliative care needs, whose needs are not best met in a non-palliative care setting. Such patients might require an acute hospital bed or they might be too sick to move to a hospice or other NHS palliative care unit. As discussed briefly at the start of this chapter, hospital income and activity is measured in (medical) consultant episodes of care and many consultant colleagues find the concept of working in a purely advisory capacity very difficult to grasp. Requests to take over a patient's care are frequent, even when a team is advisory and has no beds. Some also feel that having beds enables palliative care to be viewed on an equal footing with other specialties by making it accountable for the management of a bed or unit in line with other specialties. Some also argue that having beds might improve job satisfaction for palliative care staff in an acute setting, by enabling them to take over and more effectively manage some patients' care, thereby having more direct control over outcomes.

What is clear is that developing specialist palliative care beds in the acute setting is complex. There is some evidence from North America that specialist palliative care units in hospitals reduces average daily or episode costs (predominantly through lower costs for drug and investigations)[2,3] but no evidence that they reduce length of stay. Such units have high capital costs (particularly if predominantly developed around single, en-suite rooms rather than bays and the development of appropriate facilities for families and caregivers) and high revenue costs, particularly in terms of staffing (e.g. an increased nurse: patient ratio compared to general wards). There is no national consensus to on how to decide which patients would be appropriate for admission to hospital palliative care units (e.g. rather than hospice) or how many beds would be required for an effective, functioning unit. Concerns may also be expressed around de-skilling general hospital staff and such units may be seen as competitive by local hospices or other NHS palliative care units. Hospital Trusts, therefore, need to be convinced that the improvements in quality of care alongside potential lower average costs, outweigh the initial capital and continuing revenue costs.

Clinical governance and palliative care in the acute hospital

When managing a palliative care service there is a responsibility to ensure that governance arrangements are in place. Clinical governance is at the centre of the NHS drive to create a modern, patient-led health service, with the fundamental aim being the provision of responsive, consistent, high-quality and safe patient care.[4] Clinical governance has been defined as '*A framework through which NHS organisations are accountable for continuously improving the quality of their services and safeguarding high standards of care by creating an environment in which excellence in clinical care will flourish.*'[5]

The key elements of clinical governance are:

1. Patient, public and caregiver involvement – analysis of patient–professional involvement and interaction, and strategy, planning and delivery of care.

2. Strategic capacity and capability – planning, communication and governance arrangements, and cultural behaviour aspects.

3. Risk management – incident reporting, infection control, prevention and control of risk.

4. Staff management and performance – recruitment, workforce planning, appraisals.

5. Education, training and continuous professional development – professional re-validation, management development, confidentiality and data protection.

6. Clinical effectiveness – clinical audit management, planning and monitoring, learning through research and audit.

7. Information management – patient records etc.

8. Communication – patient and public, external partners, internal, board and organization-wide.

9. Leadership – throughout the organization, including Board, Chair and non-executive directors, chief executive and executive directors, managers and clinicians.

10. Team working – within the service, senior managers, clinical and multidisciplinary teams, and across organizations.

Seven pillars of Clinical Governance Model (NHS Clinical Governance Support Team 1999)

Traditionally, clinical governance has been described using the seven key pillars. Although it has been refined over the past few years, this approach remains an easy way to conceptualise clinical governance (see Fig. 4.1).

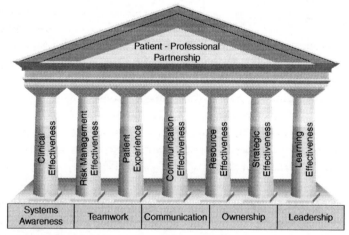

Fig. 4.1 Seven pillars of Clinical Governance Model. © NHS Clinical Governance Support Team 1999, with permission.

Clinical governance in practice

Different Trusts will have different structures in place to support clinical governance. As a team, however, you need to consider the key elements of clinical governance and put systems and processes in place to support quality improvement – such as induction and mandatory training, regular appraisal, governance meetings, a structured audit programme and effective linkage with governance structures within the Trust. It is beyond the scope of this book to discuss all aspects of clinical governance; some key factors relevant for hospital palliative care teams are discussed in the following sections.

Clinical audit

The standard definition of clinical audit, endorsed by both the National Institute of Clinical Excellence (NICE) and the Healthcare Commission, is 'Clinical audit is a quality improvement process that seeks to improve the patient care and outcomes through systematic review of care against explicit criteria and the implementation of change. Aspects of the structures, processes and outcomes of care are selected and systematically evaluated against explicit criteria. Where indicated, changes are implemented at an individual team, or service level and further monitoring is used to confirm improvement in health-care delivery'. A detailed discussion of the audit process and cycle is beyond the scope of this book but excellent generic information can be found on the NHS Clinical Governance Support Team website (*http://www.cgsupport.nhs. uk/Resources/Clinical_Audit/1@Introduction_and_Contents.asp*) and Irene Higginson's book *Clinical Audit in Palliative Care* (Radcliffe Medical Press) is a further useful resource.

Quality improvement of health services is not really possible without staff being involved in monitoring, planning, and assessing processes. Within the context of clinical governance it is essential to show that there is an evidence base to the care that is provided. Analysis of audit data enables staff to highlight areas of insufficient performance and plan improvement projects to achieve better results. A clear audit process will bring about a real improvement in patient services, and will also lead to increased competency amongst staff.

Within one of our Network areas, a robust mechanism for clinical audit has been developed. Initially formed in 1995, the audit group consists of multi-disciplinary staff working within specialist palliative care across the network area. An annual meeting takes place to decide the audit topics for the coming year. These may be regional, or local. Some are based on topics previously audited, to complete the audit cycle. A range of topics are audited – both 'clinical' and those designated as non-symptom control. Each bi-monthly meeting attracts between 50 and 60 health care professionals and begins with the presentation of a literature review around the chosen topic, followed by the results of the individual audit. An open discussion including an invited expert then takes place, which enables standards and guidelines to be developed. The guidelines are then formatted, reviewed by the group, and sent for further review by an external expert, before being disseminated.

This system has led to the development and publication of a standards and guidelines book which is now on its third edition. Care is taken to include levels of evidence within the book as demonstrated by Harbour and Miller (2001).[6] The aim of the publication from the audit cycle is to promote the setting and monitoring of standards in palliative care, and to promote clinical excellence in the care of patients whose life is drawing to a close.

Outcome measures in palliative care

In recent years, it has been seen as increasingly important to use Patient Recorded Outcome Measures (PROMS) not only in palliative care but also in all clinical specialties. This follows from a growing emphasis on the quality of the patient's experience of treatment as well as its clinical outcomes: a movement led by patients now reflected in DOH policies. Outcome measures (patient-related or not) for palliative care are problematic but it is going to be of critical importance to the specialty to able to demonstrate that palliative care services are effective in reducing patients' pain and other difficult symptoms, and improving their experience of treatment. Trusts are also interested in so-called 'invest to save' criteria such as reduced length of stay for patients or rapid discharge. If we don't have a proven positive effect, will our specialist services continue to be funded?

There are several scales for examining the outcomes of specialist palliative care interventions. These include the POS[7] and the STAS[8] and the Edmonton Symptom Assessment Scale (ESAS).[9]

In practice, we have found that when trying to evaluate our interventions, team members often find it difficult to add using a scale into their normal clinical work; they find it intrudes on establishing and building rapport and can be a distraction. Many patients are simply too ill or too distressed to fill out a self-assessment form. It is easier if you are monitoring the impact of your interventions on a specific symptom as the Breathlessness Intervention Service[10] does, where there are well-described and reasonably concise scales for this purpose, albeit limited to 'point in time' assessments rather than a measure of the global impact of the symptom. Specific scales, such as those for pain, also seem highly pertinent to the aims of the treatment when one symptom is dominant.

One approach is to ask patients to use a general symptom assessment scale (e.g. ESAS) to discern which symptom is of greatest importance and then use a specific scale to monitor progress with that symptom. Another may be to measure patients' sense of mastery of their worst symptom after specialist palliative care interventions or to use questionnaires (preferably administered by someone else as patients find it hard to believe that expressing dissatisfaction will not be found out by the team caring for them). In one of our teams, PALS are carrying out telephone evaluations of the palliative care service in outpatients and GP liaison is approaching GPs to understand their views. This approach is only the pilot stage and we do not have any data to support its use as yet.

In your setting decide what aspects of your service are most valuable to patients and referrers and then pilot an evaluation of that limited area. Use validated outcome measures delivered by someone unconnected with your service where you can, or patient-related outcome measures which can be seen to be based on patient and caregiver data only.

If you are not even trying to evaluate your service you could run into problems in the future, but there is (rightly) circumspection about the results of simple questionnaire data administered by the treating team.

Performance management of a team

It is increasingly common for Trusts to introduce structures for the performance management of clinical areas, e.g. wards, services, and divisions. The information required includes data on *objective* quality outcomes. This is likely to become universal practice and you need to consider how you would demonstrate team efficiency, financial capability, and staff capability.

In one of our organizations, this has led to the development of performance scorecards for clinical areas. In a ward, it is relatively easy to think about objective performance or quality 'targets' that can be measured (e.g. infection control, average length of stay, outpatient did not attend rates, staff compliance with appraisal or mandatory training) but this is more challenging for a palliative care team working in an advisory capacity, where most of the outcomes are qualitative rather than quantitative.

It is not possible to reproduce an example of the performance scorecard for palliative care in one of our organizations in the book but you can view it online.[1] The scorecard is divided into several sections (organizational efficiency, staff capability, and financial efficiency); in certain areas data quality is used as a proxy for targets, e.g. around organizational efficiency. In our experience, the scorecard has been useful as a way of tracking referral and contact trends (see trend graphs) and data from the scorecard has been used to support business cases for new staff. The challenge is how to evolve the scorecard so that it is more 'fit for purpose' in allowing an at-a-glance view of activity, outcomes and efficiency for the hospital team, whilst demonstrating to those

----

[1] Please note that the performance scorecard is the property of King's college Hospital NHS foundation Trust and cannot be reproduced without permission. To view please visit www.oup.com/uk/isbn/9780199238927.

outside of palliative care what it is that the service delivers. For this, further work needs to be undertaken to incorporate outcomes measures and markers of clinical complexity – for starters!

Appraisal

Regular (annual) appraisal is now a requirement for all staff working in NHS organizations and whatever the management structures for palliative care teams, all professionals within the team have a responsibility to ensure that they are appraised on a yearly basis. Where the appraisal may be undertaken by a manager who has no experience of and perhaps only limited understanding of palliative care, it may be useful to consider partnering with other organizations and undertaking joint appraisals. Although appraisal is said to be distinct from performance management, in practice it is not (see section 'Consultant appraisal') , and if you are being appraised and appraising it is wise to bear in mind that both of you will understand that this is a subtext to the meeting. The teaching that it is separate, however, may also be useful in difficult times.

The frameworks for appraisal vary between professional groups with key performance indicators (KPIs) in place for non-medical staff and formal processes for permanent doctors and those in training (see *http://www. appraisalsupport.nhs.uk/default.asp* and *https://www.appraisals.nhs.uk/*). Regular appraisal processes is one of the facets of clinical governance and compliance with appraisal is measured at a Trust level as part of the annual health check process (see *http://www.healthcarecommission.org.uk/homepage.cfm*).

If you help to manage someone of a different professional background make sure you get appropriate training in appraisal, e.g. in agenda for change KPIs, if you are a doctor helping to manage an occupational therapist.

Consultant appraisal

Consultant appraisal is now also linked to re-validation and re-licensing for doctors (for more information, see *http://www.gmcuk.org/about/reform/gmp_ framework.asp*). In summary, the GMC is preparing to introduce 'licences to practise' with periodic renewal ('revalidation'), based on positive evidence that a doctor remains up to date and fit to practise. The Government's White Paper, *Trust, Assurance and Safety – The Regulation of Health Professionals in the 21st Century*, published in February 2007, proposes that revalidation will consist of two core components: re-licensing for all doctors and specialist re-certification. Re-licensing and re-certification will depend on an objective assessment of a doctor's fitness to practise against clear standards. *Good Medical Practice* will form the basis for those standards.

Preparing for appraisal as a new consultant may seem a burdensome process, with evidence needing to be collected covering several key domains:

1. Good medical practice

2. Maintaining good medical practice

3. Managing a service

4. Teaching and training

5. Research

6. Health and probity

7. Personal effectiveness

To support this process, we have learnt that it is important to take every opportunity to collect evidence to demonstrate what you do/have achieved across these domains – whilst accepting that some of the evidence may be for the team rather than you as an individual. Collect evidence for your portfolio as you work throughout the year and immediately file in an appraisal file under the relevant headings, otherwise preparing for appraisal will be a lengthy and tedious procedure. Build this into regular practice: you will then find that although you will still need to spend time preparing for your appraisal, it is not nearly as daunting as it otherwise might have been!

Use the same technique for collecting your CPD evidence (also needed for your appraisal file) and complete your on-line diary throughout the year.

Continuing professional development

The delivery of education by the palliative care team will be dealt with in Chapter 8. However, it is imperative that each team member receives adequate opportunities to develop both clinically and intellectually. Conflict may arise amongst teams if it appears that some members are given more study time than others. Within the current climate of limited resources, study time is becoming a more precious commodity, so a sense of equality in sharing out the resources should prevail. It is important that key issues from conference attendance should be cascaded to other team members. One way of ensuring this happens is to build conference or study feedback time into team meetings. Alternatively some teams request that a brief resume of the proceedings is written and cascaded amongst all team members.

Some teams support journal clubs as a forum for sharing best practice and up to date research evidence.

In one of our services, where the clinical service works alongside a large academic palliative care department, the dissemination of information between the clinical and academic teams has been challenging. This is being addressed by a series of joint meetings: a clinical update meeting when key clinical issues or research projects are presented and discussed; and a joint journal club where journal articles with clinical and methodological relevance are presented jointly by a member of the clinical team and an academic. Such joint initiatives in larger Trusts with academic units are crucial to maintain communication between academic and clinical services to support translational and clinically relevant research.

However, in reality, most hospital teams do not have direct links with academic departments. As palliative care teams are small, it may therefore be useful to form links with local palliative care services and to share continuous professional development activities, such as journal clubs. This increases the critical mass of people involved and potentially increases the benefit by widening the expertise; this, however, needs to be balanced with the logistics of cross-site collaboration.

Consultants, associate specialist and specialist registrars in Palliative Medicine are now required to register with the Royal College of Physicians for continuing professional development. This is an online log of all educational activities undertaken, both internal and external; all activities have to be evaluated to receive 'credit'. The Royal College of Physicians has defined a minimum number of credits that have to be obtained each year; a review of CPD activity forms part of the annual appraisal and will be part of the revalidation process.

Staff in difficulty: performance management

Performance management of staff is one of the most difficult and *time-consuming* jobs of team managers. It is often the part of their role that, at least initially, keeps them awake at night feeling most isolated and alone.

The first thing to state is that it is better to prevent or intervene as early as possible with these problems than to hope they will vanish. The latter often leads to significant crises, much unpleasantness, and even when the team member is at fault they can often justifiably say that they did not know what they were doing was unsatisfactory, went on doing it and doing more of it until it became such a major issue that confrontation became unavoidable.

When a new member of staff is appointed, when someone in the team is working in a less than satisfactory way or has problems that need support or active intervention, it is imperative that you do not delay all discussion until the annual appraisal. You need to meet up as often as necessary to sort out or at least contain the effects of the issue.

New team members can set objectives after about 3 months for review in 3 months time. New team members come into a team where their work is 'not task-orientated' and where their clinical work is mostly done in conjunction with members of other teams rather than their colleagues. In such situations, it is difficult to know how one is doing or whether one is reaching expectations. Early frequent contact (it does not have to be lengthy, but it needs to be about specific issues) with a line-manager is one way of helping new staff adjust to the acute Trust. (See 'Why have you choosen to work in an acute hospital' pp 2.) This may help team members get off to the right start in their new job and helps the line-manager to assess the safety and competence of the appointee.

When you sense something is wrong or 'not quite right' there is probably something that needs attention. You then need to try and define the problem before having an early meeting to try and sort it out. Very obviously some sorts of problems (e.g. drug or alcohol abuse) brook no delay and you need support immediately but even when the problem is less weighty it can still be hard to know what to do. Do not hesitate to ask for help 'off the record' if necessary from:

1. HR or personnel: your department will probably have an assigned manager

2. Your line manager

3. Other managers involved with a problematic individual

4. A coach or supervisor

5. Books or websites concerned with personnel work

6. Your union

7. Occupational health (anonymised discussion first, asking about options)

8. And/or all of the above

You do not have to rush to formal procedures (in fact, this could be unjust) every time, but advice, off the record and anonymised if necessary, could help you formulate a way of helping.

Clinicians are often poorly trained for this aspect of their work and many prefer to overlook unhelpful behaviour in those they manage, rather than tackling it early before it becomes embedded. This can lead to much more serious problems requiring much more difficult and unpleasant management tasks than approaching the topic early on, directly with the individual concerned.

Do deal with problems early, and in a structured way (note-keeping, interviews, objectives, etc.) with support for you and the person under scrutiny. Do not expect everyone from the team to support you: you cannot divulge the problems to everyone, so individuals may tell a different story to their colleagues who may think you are being very severe. Do not be tempted to try and gain understanding by 'spin' or briefing against the individual to people outside the team who you know are not discreet. This will only amplify the problem: you need to play a long, adult game.

Do seek help as you probably are not an expert in employment law or 'good practice' in personnel work and if you handle the situation clumsily you could:

1. Make it worse
2. Split the team unnecessarily
3. Be accused of bullying
4. Have a grievance procedure taken out against you
5. Damage your confidence and then withdraw from the team
6. Regret it for the rest of your life

In summary:

1. If the problem potentially affects patient care or safety ACT IMMEDIATELY taking advice from your line manager or the individual's line manager.
2. For minor issues that could become intrusive (e.g. inappropriate jokes, erratic punctuality), act early and give specific guidance to the individual; review soon.
3. For frequent, short sick leave (e.g. more than five single days off in a year), act early: this may be stress-related.
4. For serious illness, there will be clear Trust guidance.
5. Do not expect everyone to understand and support you: find one to two people to confide in and stick to them.
6. There may be a simple reason to explain a change in behaviour/inappropriate behaviour, which can be helped (even solved) by a simple supportive action (e.g. greater flexibility in hours): find out.
7. Do not treat your colleagues as your patients or try and solve and support everything (it does not work with patients either).

Further information may be available from the National Clinical Assessment Service website *http://www.ncas.npsa.nhs.uk.*

Summary

And finally, be bold! In our experience, a positive, constructive, and helpful approach towards clinician colleagues supports integration into the hospital mainstream. We always look for opportunities to educate and promote palliative care, as many clinicians have a very narrow view of what we do. At times this can be intimidating and may involve moving well outside of one's comfort zone, taking a few risks even, but can also be very rewarding.

References

1. Department of Health (2008). End of Life Care Strategy. 8–38 (http://www.dh.gov.uk/en/Publicationsandstatistics/Publications/PublicationsPolicyAndGuidance/DH_086277).
2. Davis, M.P. et al. (2005). *J Support Oncol,* **3**, 313–316.
3. Elsayem, A. et al. (2004). *JCO,* **22**(10), 2008–2014.
4. http://www.cgsupport.nhs.uk/About_CG/default.asp.
5. Scally, G., Donaldson, L. (1998). Looking forward: clinical governance and the drive for quality improvement in the NHS in England. *BMJ,* **317**, 61–65.
6. Harbour, R., Miller, J. (2001). A new system for grading recommendations in evidence based guidelines. *BMJ,* **323**, 334–336.
7. http://www.kcl.ac.uk/schools/medicine/depts/palliative/qat/pos.html.
8. http://www.kcl.ac.uk/schools/medicine/depts/palliative/qat/stas.html.
9. http://www.palliative.org/PC/ClinicalInfo/AssessmentTools/esas.pdf.
10. Ewing, G., Farquhar, M., Booth, S. (in press). Delivering palliative care in an acute hospital setting: views of referrers and specialist providers. *J Pain Symp Manage.*

Chapter 5

Multi-disciplinary working in practice

Some definitions

It may be helpful to start with some definitions; those listed here are taken from the online Oxford English Dictionary (*http://www.askoxford.com/concise_oed*).

Multi-

Combining form more than one; many (*multi-cultural*) – Origin from Latin multus 'much, many'

Multi-disciplinary

An *adjective* involving several academic disciplines or professional specializations

Professional

1. *Adjective*: (i) relating to or belonging to a profession; (ii) engaged in an activity as a paid occupation rather than as an amateur; (iii) worthy of or appropriate to a professional person; competent.
2. *Noun*: (i) a professional person; (ii) a person having impressive competence in a particular activity.

Speciality (or specialty)

A *noun*: (i) a pursuit, area of study, or skill to which someone has devoted themselves and in which they are expert; (ii) a product for which a person or region is famous; (iii) (usu. *specialty*) a branch of medicine or surgery. Inter-specialty working therefore in this context is taken to refer to different specialty groups working together.

In the context of specialist palliative care teams the terms multi-disciplinary and multi-professional are usually used interchangeably. In this chapter we shall use the term multi-disciplinary to describe team working in palliative care.

What makes for successful teams?

There is evidence to support multi-disciplinary (or multi-professional) palliative care teams. The 2004 NICE Supportive and Palliative Care Guidance research evidence, strongly supports specialist palliative care teams working in home, hospitals, and in-patient units or hospices as a means to improve outcomes for cancer patients, such as in pain, symptom control and satisfaction, and in improving care more widely[1]. In a systematic review of the effectiveness of palliative care teams, Higginson et al report that there is a tendency for better outcomes in studies where the teams had been categorized as specialist, with multi-professional trained staff, compared to those which were nurse only, and/or had limited training[2]. In a further systematic review to determine whether teams providing specialist palliative care improve the health outcomes of patients with advanced cancer and their families or carers when compared to conventional services, Hearn and Higginson reported that the evidence indicates that a multi-professional approach with specialist input is beneficial[3]. The authors comment that the results support the use of specialist multi-professional team in palliative care to improve satisfaction of patients with advanced cancer and their family. The evidence from this review suggests that multi-professional teams were more able to identify and deal with patient / family needs, and provided access to other services.

Most of us working in specialist palliative care have been drawn to the specialty in part, by the fact that we are mostly working in multi-disciplinary teams (MDTs). Whilst this can at times be challenging (see next section), the positives usually far outweigh the negatives. Some of the key positives of working in MDTs are outlined below:

Key benefits of MDT working

1. Ability to learn from other professionals in the team.
2. Team members bring different background and skill sets usually enabling the sum of the whole to be greater than the individual parts.

---

[1] National Institute for Clinical Excellence. Improving Supportive & Palliative Care for Adults with Cancer. *http://www.nice.org.uk/guidance/index.jsp?action=byID&o=10893# documents*.

[2] Higginson IJ, Finlay IG, Goodwin DM, Hood K, Edwards AGK, Cook A et al. Is there evidence that palliative care teams alter end-of-life experiences of patients and their caregivers? *Journal of Pain & Symptom Management*, 2003;25: 150–68.

[3] Hearn J,. Higginson IJ. Do specialist palliative care teams improve outcomes for cancer patients? A systematic literature review. *Palliat Med*, 1998;12: 317–32.

3. Professionals with different training and background often see the world differently, enabling a real mix of skills in dealing with patients and families.

4. No one individual has all the skills it takes to deliver effective palliative care but a team may have.

5. Mutual support.

6. Ability to share out the workload and support each other in dealing with challenging patients and families.

7. It can be really helpful and supportive to discuss difficult problems with a team member – to offer new ideas and to support you when there are no easy answers.

8. It's great fun.

Challenges of multi-disciplinary working

Whilst MDTs deliver the best outcomes for patients and families, in practice they can be challenging to work in. In the UK in most hospital palliative care teams, there are different management structures in place for different team members and this has the potential to lead to a lack of shared vision and ownership of a team and, at worst, the development of a 'them and us' culture.

As outlined in Chapter 2, the NICE guidance on supportive and palliative care describes a core team of a (medical) consultant, clinical nurse specialist, and administrator. In most palliative care MDTs with a medical consultant in place, he/she will act as the clinical lead for the team, directly linking in to hospital Trust management structures and will represent the team both internally and externally. Larger hospital teams may also have a nursing team leader, who may have line management responsibility for non-medical team members and who will represent the team from a nursing perspective within the hospital Trust. These dual management structures have the potential to lead to miscommunication and lack of a shared sense of direction and ownership for the team, which can be challenging to team dynamics.

Many hospital palliative care teams now also have specialist psychosocial support, with the appointment of psychologists and social workers to form truly multi-professional teams. However, whilst the doctors and nurses in palliative care MDTs may fit easily into hospital Trust management structures, in our experience there may be few psychosocial staff in acute hospital Trusts and they can feel isolated both within a team (as a professional of one in a team with other, larger professional groups) and within the wider organization.

Team dynamics may also be challenged by personality differences. Within a team some individuals may be more confident or extrovert than others and great care needs to be taken that these people do not dominate the team unhealthily. In our experience of working in small teams, any issue (real or perceived) can easily be magnified in a context where the working relationships are so intense, leading to dissatisfaction amongst team members which can be very damaging in the medium and long term. It is inevitable that at times team members will disagree with each other – what is really key is the team dynamic in which they occur and how they are managed.

Space – or a lack of it – may also contribute to difficulties within teams. Any issues may be exacerbated by cramped working conditions and some team members may feel claustrophobic within confined office accommodation.

All of the issues highlighted above may lead to different team members feeling isolated or without an equal voice. This can result in tensions that may be poorly understood by other team members. In order to avoid conflicts escalating and to maintain a shared vision for the team, it is crucial that the clinicians communicate regularly, openly, and honestly.

In our experience several strategies may help to promote healthy team dynamics:

1. Regular team meetings to promote open communication.

2. In large teams, regular meetings with senior team members (e.g. medical consultant, lead nurse, senior psychosocial specialist) to promote shared vision for development of team and service delivery.

3. Welcome lunches and/or drinks for new team members.

4. Try to make time for stopping for a team coffee or lunch at least once a month – and try to ensure that this happens away from the office.

5. Allow people 'time out' of team collective activities, e.g. eating lunch with colleagues outside the team or on their own in the canteen instead in the team office, leaving early after a 'bad patch' with very demanding clinical work.

6. Social events can be particularly successful when focused around an activity (so potentially everyone can make a fool of themselves)!

7. Consider team building sessions if required – these sessions can work (see Chapters 2 and 10 for more information)! If team dynamics have become so strained that you are considering team building, sourcing an external facilitator is crucial – a good facilitator is neutral and will have the skills to pull the team together and facilitate communication.

Clinical versus other activities

One of the key tensions that can arise is that senior staff have responsibilities that are beyond clinical. For example, a palliative medicine consultant job plan will have time allocated to clinical activities (e.g. attendance at MDMs, ward rounds, clinics, patient administration) and time for 'supporting professional activities (SPAs)' – these activities include teaching, training, clinical governance, research, and management (see Chapter 2 for more information on consultant job plans). More senior consultants may have responsibilities that will take them off site frequently – for Network, Deanery, or Royal College activities, for example. Senior nurse specialists, e.g. team leaders, or nurse consultants, will also have non-clinical responsibilities, including management, teaching, and training and again these activities may require them to be off-site for periods of time.

Indeed Cicely Saunders' vision for modern palliative care was that of excellence in clinical care, alongside teaching and research to inform practice. Therefore, for all staff working in palliative care there is a need to balance delivering clinical care and training generalist staff by teaching and training programmes and getting involved in research where possible. This need to balance activities inevitably causes tensions: the patient and family needs are often immediate and real, but forever prioritizing clinical activity over other activities leads to services stagnating, not developing and ultimately not providing the best, evidence-based care.

In our experience, more junior team members may not always understand the competing demands placed on more senior team members and may end up feeling resentful and unsupported; senior team members also may not effectively communicate with the team and may feel that the pressures they are under are not acknowledged.

We cannot pretend to have all the answers to these issues but open and effective communication is paramount. One of us, in a team that has recently grown significantly in size, has found the use of a white board weekly diary, a helpful starting point to outline where team members are, what they are doing and to highlight potential times in the week when the service may be stretched.

Working with other specialties

Inter-specialty working is the cornerstone of successful hospital palliative care teams. Without interacting with professional groups across the organization, teams will become isolated and will not be able to build and develop. Many people working in palliative care are drawn to the hospital setting not only to work in a larger organization but because of the opportunity to interact with multiple specialty groups. Whilst this in inherently challenging, it is also fun and rewarding, promoting an atmosphere of continual learning and development of a broad range of skills.

As described elsewhere in this book, however, hospital palliative care teams are very small cogs in the large, complex systems that are hospitals. For palliative care teams to be successful they have to tread a careful line – of being helpful and supportive to other clinical teams in order to obtain referrals and thereby to effectively manage patients with palliative care problems, whilst promoting the specialty of palliative care, educating the generalists (in practice non-palliative care specialists who may feel that they 'know best') and working in an advocacy role for patients and families. In order for this tightrope to be successfully negotiated, most of the time, excellent communication, diplomacy, and negotiation skills are required. In our experience, most hospital palliative care teams are valued and respected, but such successful inter-specialty working requires a specific skill set, time, and patience.

Here are a few helpful hints to optimize inter-specialty working:

1. Be approachable and try to maintain a 'can-do' mentality.

2. Make the referral process as straightforward as possible – easy access is crucial; try to avoid the referral process becoming a barrier.

3. Ensure that teams know how to access the palliative care team – and that hours of working are clear – to minimize accusations of inaccessibility.

4. Working in an advisory role can be frustrating – try to think of it as a partnership between teams, with the optimal outcomes for patients as the priority. It is also useful to remember that the specialists you are working alongside may know the patients well and will bring invaluable specialist knowledge – palliative care will not have all the answers. Therefore, when agreeing management plans, a constructive dialogue and negotiation with the specialist team that the patient is under is likely to be very helpful in agreeing a way forward.

5. Try to keep frustrations under wraps, especially when your advice appears to be disregarded or ignored. It is much better to lose your rag back in the safety of your office rather than on the ward, where you can be sure that ward staff will remember!

6. Diplomacy and negotiation are key – over time, you'll need your best communication skills! (see section 'Negotiating skills' below)

7. Many specialists that you are working with may not really understand palliative care (let alone really know what it is) – but you may also not really understand their specialty skills and knowledge. It is easy to get defensive – try to avoid this and whilst being helpful and charming, try to gently educate and inform.

8. It is useful to keep in mind that advisory palliative care teams are playing a long game – it is better to lose a few battles but to overall win the war.

Working in an advisory role in hospital palliative care is not for the faint-hearted and you will find that good communication and negotiation skills are crucial. For this reason, we have outlined some key facets underpinning effective negotiation in the next section.

Negotiating skills

What are negotiating skills?

In clinical and strategic work it is normal for different people, specialists in their own right, to have different opinions about the best way forward in easy and difficult situations. When handled correctly, this is helpful because the combination of two approaches or mixed strategies taken from different stand-points or disciplines will usually offer the patient and the team a number of valuable ways forward. Disagreement, or to use a more loaded word conflict, is only unhelpful and even destructive when clinical or strategic decisions become tangled up in personal or interpersonal doubts, insecurities, and concerns. Developing or improving already existing negotiating skills is an absolute essential for anyone who wants to give the best care to patients or develop and drive forward an effective strategy for their service or specialty. Giving excellent clinical care now requires effective team work and collaboration between different clinical teams. It is, of course, still true that carrying out an excellent operation, doing an excellent pain consultation, or helping an individual family sort out their psychosocial problems to the highest standard, may be the activity or remit of one individual – but increasingly, good outcomes require effective teamwork.

Most clinicians say that their greatest pleasure comes from their work with their patients and their greatest worries or sense of despondency comes from their work with either the NHS 'system' or the individuals within it. When we negotiate, we are trying to achieve, by discussion, an agreement on an area where two or more parties will receive different benefits or outcomes from an activity. There are many examples of negotiation from everyday life and clinical practice, e.g. the price of something, the best way to conduct clinical care, the next strategic priority, resources to be allotted to a project, and so on. As clinicians working in advisory roles, negotiation becomes part of everyday life.

It has been said so often that it is now a cliché, that negotiation should ideally be conducted with the idea of achieving an outcome that pleases all parties equally. This is often called, inelegantly, a 'win-win' situation. Some compromises seem to be based on the idea of equal displeasure for all parties: such agreements rarely last.

The idea of a 'win-win agreement' has become a cliché because it is the most desirable outcome for negotiations. Everyone needs to be able to support important agreements genuinely, perhaps with reservations and regrets, but whole-heartedly, because otherwise the greatest strategy and the most effective care pathway, the most subtle and ambitious clinical care plan, can be subverted consciously or unconsciously by disgruntled participants who may give every outward appearance of engagement.

When does negotiation take place in a palliative care service?

You are conducting many, many negotiations big and small every day in the course of your working and private life. When both of you reach the doorway at the same time, you negotiate, usually automatically and unthinkingly, who should go first; you negotiate who is going to do what in a team, when you take your lunch, what sort of work you can get done in the time available in the course of the day, which work you need to do first. You have already developed, if you have longstanding friends and agreeable colleagues, some effective negotiation strategies. Let's see what these entail.

Seeing the bigger picture

When you both arrive at the doorway at the same time, if you both try and walk through together or at the same time in opposite directions, you will both be hindered, possibly injured. If you agree to do more work than is possible in one day, you will be at least in the longer term, resentful, stressed, worn down, eventually ineffective, and either resign or be fired. If you refuse outright with no explanation and a very harsh way, to do work that comes within your remit, although not possible in the timeframe given, you will also damage your reputation. If this happens consistently, it will lead to bad feeling, dissatisfaction with your work, and perhaps in the long term, the loss of your job. The reason this doesn't happen is because you jointly or separately see the way to a productive outcome, even if this means giving way with good grace or accepting some small temporary disadvantage with good humour, for longer term greater gains. Both (or all of you) will benefit from a better longer-term outcome of a successful cohesive team where work is shared than would be possible if you both held to very rigid interpretation of what was best for you immediately or at all times.

You all offer something

Sometimes you will not see that the other party has given anything and you may have to 'rise above' some residual anger if, for example, you have to stop your car at a 'give way' sign when it was really your right of way. In these circumstances you have given way because the consequences of sticking rigidly to what is 'legal' or 'right' are so serious that it is not worth not compromising.

On the other hand, the situation may be so trivial that it is silly not to give way, e.g. letting someone barge through the door in front of you. Even so you can still be left feeling resentful or bemused and disappointed, at the least.

On important and major issues you cannot have a really successful negotiation which leads to sustainable long-term and long-lasting changes with advantage to all, if parties have not contributed something, even if it is only their goodwill and commitment to support a new way of doing things.

Exploration of all the possibilities takes place first

With all sorts of negotiations which are important in hospital palliative care, it is crucial that assumptions about the range of possible outcomes are not too narrow, that everyone is prepared to think more widely than their normal practice. In the bigger negotiations in which you will take part, the most difficulty occurs when you have two parties or teams or individuals with diametrically opposed, fixed alternative options. If ever you find yourself going to the negotiating table or are in negotiation and you think that it can only be your chosen action or the other's chosen action which can take place without alteration, you are probably entering very difficult territory and unlikely to reach agreement. Let's look at an apparently 'either or' clinical choice: this case study will be used to illustrate aspects of negotiation skills.

Case study: Mr T

You are called urgently to the haematology outpatient clinic. Mr T is a 32 -year -old man with advanced Hodgkin's lymphoma. You have been asked to see him because of his severe psychological distress. When you arrive, he is in tears, almost shaking with grief, his distraught partner (mother of their 3 -year old and 18 -month -old children) is trying to comfort him. The haematologist has said there is no further treatment (he means chemotherapy) available. Mr T tells you he thinks he has been 'sentenced to death'. When you go to talk to the haematology consultant privately, he says it would be unethical to offer this man any other chemotherapy as it would (a) not work, (b) possibly do him harm. You tell him that Mr T had told you about a unit in a neighbouring city where they would offer him a mixture of steroids and 5-fluorouracil (5-FU), you both know that it will not do anything to either cure the disease or even prolong his life, but it may help him emotionally and has few adverse effects.

Possible solutions:
1. See that the haematologist has the patient's best interests at heart. The haematologist is actually taking a pure moral and ethical stand based on medical evidence. His grounds for wanting to deny the patient further chemotherapy are based on his view of the patient's best interests and his duty to prescribe treatment according to the best available evidence in the literature and on a completely logical standpoint.

2. Your favoured management plan after further lengthy discussions with the patient and the partner, both alone and separately, is that Mr T cannot accept that there is 'nothing' more that can be done for him. He feels it is unacceptable when he has two young children and a wife who are completely financially dependent on him. He does not want to 'give up' without a fight and fighting to him means chemotherapy and active treatment. They understand that the other unit is not offering a cure or even a guaranteed prolongation of his life, but they want to explore the option so they feel as a family they are doing everything they can to go on living as a family.

This sort of distressing situation is where feelings can run high. Some palliative care clinicians might feel it was their duty to dissuade him from seeking further chemotherapy and that he was not 'coming to terms' with his illness. They then have to negotiate this with the patient. An alternative view is that the patient and family's instinct of what was best for them, which would not harm other people, would not incur huge extra crippling expense, denying other people treatment could possibly be of both short- and longer-term psychological benefit to the family and for the rest of that patient's life. This would weigh more than the purely 'disease-focused' approach.

The wrong way to negotiate

In the course of your second discussion with the patient you start to become more and more angry, feeling that this haematologist, who is new to the Trust but who has had a 'run-in' with one of your team colleagues, and who has a brusque and apparently uncaring manner, is in the *wrong*. You demand to see him again while he's still seeing another patient and in the strongest possible terms tell him he's got to change his mind and if he doesn't, you're going to be 'the patient's advocate', go to his Clinical Director if necessary to 'fight' for the patient's rights. You then remind him of the encounter that your colleague has already had with him when you think he was coming to his rescue in a difficult situation on the haematology ward but where he was apparently patronizing. A shouting match in the side room ensues; raised voices are then heard in the clinic room which is next door to where the patient and his partner are sitting. Clinical stalemate ensures you have two angry clinicians who will probably never refer patients to each other again and an immediate impasse in the patient's management.

A possibly more productive strategy

Don't feel it beneath your dignity to wait until the haematologist has finished talking to the patient he is seeing: you may be able to meet with the specialist haematology nurse about your concerns in the meantime and phone the GP to find more information from them while you're waiting. You need to alert the GP to what has happened as he hasn't seen the patient for several months while he's been undergoing intensive treatment, (he now knows that the district nurse and health visitor and himself need to be involved). When you go in to speak to the consultant with the specialist nurse there, you explore your viewpoint that the palliative chemotherapy may be helpful for the patient in a psychological sense, and is unlikely to do harm. The haematologist is initially surprised as he thought palliative medicine was all about stopping treatments like chemotherapy and 'letting nature take its course', the patient being surrounded at that point by a number of kind but largely ineffectual clinicians. You sense this picture of the specialty but don't bridle or take offence, continue on with your favoured plan which would support the patient being referred to this other unit with the proviso that Mr T clearly understands this is for specialist palliative care intervention, not a cure of his illness. You explain that you have discussed with the patient's family that they will now be well served by having involvement with the specialist team in the community. This would gradually move the focus of care to palliation and prepare for end-of-life care, though you do not make this explicit. It also stops a rather brutal disengagement with the haematology unit over a short period when he has known them for some years. You will negotiate with the community team who are separate organization from you in a town some 30 miles away and see if they will offer blood transfusions. You will then start to negotiate with the patient and family the criteria, indications for antibiotics, and other supportive treatments (which he fears he will lose) and the circumstances under which he will be re-admitted to the haematology ward: the haematologists would have wanted him admitted as an outlier if he were to be unwell. Make it clear to the haematologist that it may take a while for this to be acceptable to him as he will need to have gained confidence in the community palliative care service and his GP before losing contact with his own specialist haematology unit.

Later, when this particular situation has settled (and possibly your strategy has allowed the family to adjust), you catch up with the haematologist who says how hard he finds it 'letting people "particularly young people" die', but that he feels he needs to be honest with people when he can't do anything. You agree to come and talk to the haematology unit on communication skills and difficult conversations making a mental note to make it clear, without reference to the individual, that phrases such as 'there's nothing we can do' are generally unhelpful as they're both inaccurate (there's always specialist palliative care) and frightening for the patient, as well as making them feel they're somehow not worth 'the effort or money involved in modern treatments'.

With the second approach or something like it, although you've probably invested a couple of hours of time and demonstrated enormous self-restraint in the face of poor understanding and initial low rating of your specialty, you have probably gained the respect and confidence of both parties. Your aim is to bring about, in the future, a more anticipatory approach to the needs of haematological patients (a specialty where it is common for sudden transitions from active treatment to specialist palliative care) and this will result in long-term benefits to other haematology patients with specialist palliative care needs.

Useful pointers

In the course of a negotiation both those that are protracted and those taking place in the course of a conversation, be aware of the following in yourself:

1. Feelings of anger either about something the other party has said or about past encounters with that person or team which have left you with unfinished business.

2. Feelings of self-righteousness: suppress them at that moment and scrutinize these feelings at a later date when you are not feeling so emotionally charged.

3. The desire to see the other person or party 'thwarted', diminished, or humiliated (as they have done to you) and this episode seems to offer you a wonderful opportunity.

If there is any strong negative emotion attached to your negotiation and if you don't experience feelings of relief and satisfaction, as you work towards a mutual productive outcome, be on your guard. You may be about to sabotage something which would benefit not only you and your service but also innocent parties like patients who deserve and require high professional standards from you. These standards involve you putting personal animosity to one side.

If you do consistently allow personal feelings and pre-occupations to interfere with clinical care or negotiations with other teams or individuals, this behaviour in time will become noticed by the wider clinical community who will lose respect and trust in you. In the longer term this could have devastating professional consequences as behaviour like this tends to escalate if unchecked; leaving aside the effects on your service and your colleagues. Unfortunately, clinical managers are often slow to address personal foibles or faults as these conversations are so difficult. If such conversations were carried out early, the need for a clinician to get their own way all the time would be less likely to develop into a potentially damaging, even dangerous habit. Learn to know yourself: if you develop a reputation for implacability, aggression, arrogance, intolerance, or even self-righteousness and bullying, at some point there may be an episode which acts as a flashpoint requiring action at the highest level and your career may even end prematurely, mired in controversy.

Negotiation and compromise are necessary professional skills: knowing when you should not compromise and should stick to your guns, without alienating people on personal grounds, is the obverse of this.

Strategic negotiations

Often strategic negotiations are a process which may seem almost interminable and therefore a long-term project rather than an episode. That's why it is so important for your team/department to conduct strategic planning (see section below). If you do not have such discussions within your team in which you plan the way ahead over a period of months or years, although you will not notice any problems in the short term (as you would if you failed to see patients, or answer letters or emails in a timely way), in the longer term your service will suffer because there's no sense of direction or drive and no ability to respond to opportunities for funding or support, which sometimes arise at the most unusual times. Palliative care services have to be nothing if not opportunistic if they are to thrive and develop as funding does not come easily to them.

When you are planning a strategic negotiation, there are several factors to consider:

1. Decide what you hope to achieve.

2. Agree some achievement milestones.

3. Decide what the service change or development will look like when it's complete, then break the journey to reach this goal into small steps.

4. Decide at which fora service developments are most likely to be taken forward and where they need to be heard.

5. Decide who the best people or teams that you need to enlist for support both inside the Trust and outside either from community palliative care teams, locality groups, the strategic health authority, or nationally recognized leaders in, for example, the 'end of life care strategy'. If there's only one of you in a management role, it's easy to see who's going to take forward the team's strategy. If you're fortunate enough to have colleagues, a consultant, a senior nurse, perhaps even an AHP specialist or psychologist or social worker working with you, divide up the strategic work into areas of interest or meetings that people are already attending as part of their work to take the strategy forward in that arena.

Stage 1

It is as important to decide who is/are the most effective team member(s) to take a strategy forward as deciding the objectives of the strategy. If the consultant has had difficulty working with a particular individual, but the senior nurse gets on well with them, as long as it is not an attempt at 'divide and rule' from outside the team, the senior nurse may be the one who's best placed to take this particular strategic initiative forward. Sometimes cross-professional negotiations are better. Consultants may be particularly irked by other consultants, nurses by other nurses and although you may feel that it's more important to rise above these feelings, sometimes it is also important to recognize when it's just easier and not inappropriate to go with the flow and match people who are effective with each other rather than connecting members of the same profession or group.

Designing your fall back point

Whatever you're negotiating, even if it's clear that everyone has to give something, it's not right if someone, or one team, has to give everything. Therefore, it's particularly unhelpful if you put all your negotiating cards on the table at the first meeting. You also need to anticipate possible blocks to the success of your strategic negotiation (who may lose by it and therefore oppose it?) and work out what the range of possibilities is in order to identify inventive, constructive, and creative ways round barriers. Don't assume what the blocks are; and don't assume that you know other people's attitudes or assumptions before you've explored them. They may well have changed since the last time you talked to them, perhaps because of an internal discussion within their own team, the effect of a national initiative, something that's happened with a patient which points out the usefulness of what you are planning, or even because life's got better for them in general and they don't feel so vigilant about everything happening around them.

Stage 2

If the issue is potentially controversial, arrange a meeting on neutral ground and leave a good gap of time in your diary between it and the preceding activity, so that you can get there before the meeting starts in an unflustered way. Be well prepared with any notes or agreements from the team that you have decided beforehand or minutes from previous meetings. If you feel there is likely to be some hostility or unpleasantness, try and go with someone else from your team who is confident to speak out and who can see the problem from the point of view of a different professional group. You may even go with someone from another department who shares your view and would be affected by the change. Canvassing people before meetings at other venues, e.g. lunch or in the corridor, if done in the right way and in the right spirit, may be a useful way of learning how other people feel before you put your proposal or for getting useful feedback and uncovering opposition or concerns where you didn't know it existed. Blatantly trying to pressurize people into supporting you at a meeting simply because you want them to is not a good plan, as people do not like to feel manipulated or used.

In summary

Stage 1

If you want to get a difficult, controversial new or radical idea through, take it slowly, give people time to adjust by presenting it at different fora in an exploratory way rather than 'we must do this way' beforehand. Put feelers out to different individuals whose opinion and knowledge you respect and who work in different departments to your own. Be prepared to modify at this stage. Marshall your facts, not your personal feelings about the proposed change and ensure you have tried to see the effects for other teams and individuals.

Even if it is a simple, to your mind, straightforward initiative (e.g. the appointment of a Macmillan specialist nurse), take nothing for granted and make sure you prepare in the same way.

You are likely to get things achieved more quickly if:

1. There is a government target to be met at all costs e.g. the waiting time guidance for A&E encouraged many Trusts to employ more consultants.

2. You have money behind you – perhaps from a major charity or, more rarely, from a benefactor.

Find out who else outside your Trust might support your idea – think of the Strategic Health Authority, NICE guidance, Royal College guidance (the latter are not always popular so choose your outside supporters carefully, especially if you are considering the PCT).

Many palliative care innovations have been supported by Macmillan Cancer Support (including the teams in which the authors work); their policy of pump-priming individuals within Trusts on the proviso that the PCT or hospital would guarantee to continue the funding at the end of the period of support, led to the foundation of many hospital teams.

Macmillan Cancer Support has changed its policies now, but it is always worth talking to your local area Macmillan manager to see if your idea falls in with the organizations current strategy. You could use the 'pump-priming' method if you can find monies from other charities or even from money your team has been given or earned from education, etc. Having something to bring to the table that you are willing to commit yourself is very powerful.

Stage 2

When you're presenting a new strategy which is potentially controversial, make sure you've identified advantages to people outside your own team or patient group. This is usually relatively easy in palliative care as most of our strategies are designed to benefit patients with any disease at a particular phase in their lives.

Stage 3: Deal with criticism

Listen carefully to criticism, some of it may be true and some of it will be helpful in the longer run. Do however, have your antennae attuned to detect criticism that may be:

1. Personally directed although disguised as a criticism of your idea. Make sure you don't identify it as your sole idea but as one that has been consulted on widely and therefore is seen as beneficial by a number of individuals and teams.

2. Ignorance: from people who have no idea about the remit for palliative care. In this case do not get angry and defensive or critical; simply state the FACTS of your case and how it fits in with nationally agreed standards such as the NICE guidance, or the end-of-life care strategy.

3. Designed to frustrate a strategy that another department or person finds threatening.

If it falls into these categories, deal with it indirectly rather than head on (i.e. do not resort to 'ad hominen' arguments or pointing out what the protagonist is doing) as this may fossilize your opposing positions.

Steadily, patiently keep promoting the facts.

When you do not get what you hoped

Most strategic negotiations take months, even years. Therefore, do not get despondent if you do not get what your service requires quickly. Re-group and re-think with your colleagues.

Ask yourselves:

1. How important is this initiative?

2. How important is it that it goes ahead?

3. Why does it need to go ahead?

4. Should trying to continue with this initiative take priority over others or would giving it a rest for few months and taking something else forward be the best move?

5. Who else/where else (NICE guidance, Trust strategies) could give you support?

6. Can you identify anything you could do better or differently next time?

Summary

Multi-disciplinary (MD) working is central to effective palliative care and the concept is particular to the specialty. It means more than a number of individuals from different backgrounds working within their own profession or specialty alongside each other in the care of one patient. In a hospital palliative care service, MD working is even more crucial than in a hospice, as there will be little understanding of what it entails from outside the team. It is essential to invest time and energy in making it work.

Chapter 6

Bureaucracy and money

NHS structure in relation to acute hospitals[1]

There are 290 NHS Hospital Trusts which oversee 1600 NHS hospitals and specialist care centres. They are commissioned to provide services by primary care trusts and, for some specialist services, locality commissioning groups of strategic health authorities. Foundation trusts are a newer type of NHS hospital of which are currently 92 available across England. In addition, there are (after re-organization in 2006) 10 Strategic Health Authorities (SHAs), organized on a regional basis, which have the responsibility of co-ordinating the strategies of the health trusts in their regions.

Healthcare Commission[2]

The Healthcare Commission is the independent watchdog for health care in England, which is responsible for assessing and reporting on the performance of both NHS and independent health care organizations to ensure that they are providing a high standard of care. It promotes continuous improvement in the services provided by the NHS and independent health care organizations.

Acute Trusts

Hospitals are managed by acute Trusts, which ensure that hospitals provide high-quality health care, and that they spend their money efficiently. They are not trusts in the legal sense but are in effect public sector corporations. Each Trust is headed by a board consisting of executive and non-executive directors and is chaired by a non-executive director. Non-executive directors are recruited by open advertisement. All NHS Trust Boards are required to have an Audit Committee consisting only of non-executive directors, on which the Chairman may not sit. This committee is entrusted not only with supervision of financial audit, but of systems of corporate governance within the Trust.

---

[1] http://www.nhs.uk/aboutnhs/HowtheNHSworks/authoritiesandtrusts/Pages/authoritie-sandtrusts.aspx#q01.

[2] http://www.healthcarecommission.org.uk/homepage.cfm.

Foundation Trusts

NHS Foundation Trusts are a fundamental part of the current NHS reform programme in the UK, reflecting the move from a centrally managed service towards the one that is managed locally and so more responsive to patients. Foundation trusts have been given much more financial and operational freedom than other NHS Trusts but remain within the NHS and its performance inspection system. They were first introduced in April 2004, and there are now 92 foundation Trusts in England.

NHS Foundation Trusts are:[3]

1. A new type of NHS organization, established as independent public benefit corporations
2. Free from central government control and from strategic health authority performance management
3. Providers of health care according to core NHS principles – free care, based on need and not on ability to pay
4. Accountable to local people, who can become members and governors
5. Free to innovate for the benefit of their local community and patients
6. Able to decide for themselves what capital investment is needed in order to improve their services
7. Free to retain any surpluses they generate and to borrow in order to support this investment
8. Authorised and monitored by Monitor - Independent Regulator of NHS Foundation Trusts

Whilst Foundation Trusts were set up to enable hospitals to have 'more freedom' than is usual for hospitals, many of these freedoms have been curtailed or have been rarely used to date (for example, being allowed to opt out of national terms and conditions of employment).

The structure of Foundation Trusts is modelled on private companies; for example they have a board of managers with executive and non-executive directors. They also have patient, community, and staff governors who can have some impact on policy. The non-executive directors are drawn from the local community and are usually appointed because they have a range of skills the Trust wants within the organization. In this regard, there are similarities with hospice Trustees.

The Chief Executive has overall responsibility for delivering the organization's strategy, but the Chair is often the most powerful person, overseeing the

[3] *http://www.monitor-nhsft.gov.uk/register_nhsft.php.*

strategic direction of the Trust and having a key role in appointing the Chief Executive, Medical Director, and the non-executives ('non-execs'). The Chair and non-executives have to ensure that the Trust acts ethically, responsibly and are expected to raise concerns about strategy where they feel it is straying from these parameters. They are also responsible for looking out for misconduct or impropriety on the part of directors of the Trust or mis-management of any sort of the organization.

Working within NHS management structures

The structure of each Trust (whether an acute Trust or a Foundation Trust) differs slightly, but it is important that you know:

1. The Trust management structure pertinent to your organization.
2. Who the Chief Executive, the Chair, and non-executive directors are.
3. The different areas, roles, and responsibilities for each director.
4. Your Trust's overall strategic direction and priorities so that these can be referred to in your business plans, bids, initiatives, etc.

Understanding the structures in which you work is crucial for developing your service. Any strategy development and/or implementation is more likely to be successful if it is not divorced from that of the rest of the Trust. You will usually find one non-executive director who has a particular interest in palliative care; if there isn't one you may suggest that someone takes on this responsibility. In large Trusts it is unlikely that you will know what is going on in other departments without regular contact with someone on the board: this enables you to make alliances with other clinicians and managers with whom you can share initiatives (e.g. education) or applications for funding. This makes applications or initiatives stronger and more likely to succeed if they cross boundaries within the Trust and have multiple champions in every department. Ensure you are aware of Trust activity at board level.

Every time the Chief Executives or Chair changes, it is worth arranging to meet the new incumbent. Merely arranging a meeting is pretty pointless; there is no rush, so it is best to go when you have something you want or need to say, or where you feel they may be helpful to the service or because you think your service is doing something noteworthy. There is nothing worse than a meeting without an agenda and it is good practice that you have one for any meeting, therefore:

1. Have an agenda, it helps to focus your mind, and if you cannot write one don't meet.
2. Send any brief backing documents (not thousands of attachments) before hand, focusing on the area of greatest interest.

3. Outline one or two key points that you want to cover in that meeting.

4. Afterwards record any agreements from the meeting in bullet points and send them back by email. If it is inappropriate to send meeting points for whatever reason, do make sure that you keep a record for yourself, filing them on the computer system in a retrievable way.

5. You may also want to keep duplicate paper records of any meeting, then your PA or administrative staff can access them in the office if you are away (in addition, if they are mislaid, there will always be a copy available).

It is very important that any strategy you wish to take forward within or without the Trust gathers support right from the beginning. It is sometimes possible to alienate people by going about it in the wrong way. If you take an issue, concern, or strategy directly to Board level without having signalled this in someway within your own Directorate, your clinical director may think you are trying to bypass them, which is not a good idea. On the other hand you do not have to always ask permission to approach the board, so do go with your ideas; just make sure you cannot be misinterpreted.

Working strategically with your organization

In building a successful service, it is not only important for you to understand the context in which you are working but also to be up to date with local, regional, and national initiatives. Working strategically outside of your organization is covered in subsequent sections in this chapter.

In our experience, there are several factors that will facilitate developing your service:

1. Keep your eyes and ears open to any local initiatives that potentially offer you an opportunity for service development, especially if this fits with the strategic direction of the Trust.

2. Ensure that you engage with any strategy work within your organization and outside of it – if you are not part of shaping services, it will happen without you and you may miss out on resources.

3. In smaller teams, you may feel that you have to drive changes yourself. However, it is crucial that you engage other team members and keep them appraised of any opportunities for development: use them to brainstorm ideas and to ensure that ideas are workable in practice.

4. In a larger team you may have the staff to develop a management team – of consultants, senior nurse(s), and other senior clinicians. Ensure that such a group has a link to representation from your divisional management team.

5. Try to develop effective working relationships with your Divisional management team – they can help you to develop your management skills

and do much of the leg-work in helping shape your ideas into a realistic business case.

6. Try to push against open rather than closed doors – so, take advantage of opportunities that present themselves and develop key allies to support you.

7. Try to start to think strategically.

   i. What are the current strengths and weaknesses of our service? What are the gaps?

   ii. What are the existing opportunities for development?

   iii. What is happening locally and regionally?

   iv. Are there any relevant national strategies that can support service developments?

   v. What is the local Trust context – in terms of strategy and how palliative care can fit into that?

   vi. Where do we want to be in 1, 2, and 5 years time?

   vii. What do we need to get there?

   viii. What opportunities are there for securing funding for service developments?

Developing business cases

Where applying for local, regional or national funding, you are likely to have to write a business case. So is there a key to successful business cases? The authors can not pretend to have all the answers here, having written many unsuccessful ones in their time, but a few pointers for potential success are outlined as follows:

1. Be really clear what it is you are asking for and what the benefit will be for the organization.

2. Think about outlining what palliative care is about (in one or two sentences) to give some context for your bid – as many readers will not really know.

3. What evidence can you provide to support your proposal? You are likely to need to provide some relevant background information and may well need to reference national publications (e.g. Department Health end-of-life care strategy 2008; national service frameworks) in addition to providing local data (e.g. from activity data, audits) to support your bid.

4. Be able to clearly articulate your current position and the potential risks associated with this.

5. Be able to outline how local, network, and national strategies fit with your proposed development – if your proposal does not fit any local or national

priorities, then it is very unlikely to get funded (so make sure that you have seen your Trust and directorate's strategies; if you have your own team strategy, reference that; also take into account national drivers, e.g. end-of-life care and the network palliative care strategy – you have to try to be savvy and may need to fit your ideas around others' strategic drivers).

6. Make sure you get your costings right, including on costs for staff and add in any equipment costs that are anticipated (e.g. computers) – these are so-called 'start-up' costs

7. If you are looking at pick up funding for a post that will initially be pump primed by an outside agency, e.g. Macmillan Cancer Support, ensure that you are clear how long the funding is for and when the Trust needs to take on the costs. Ensure this is all water tight. Macmillan Cancer Support will require Chief Executive support for any bid and the subsequent financial agreement will commit the Trust to pick up funding – however, you will need to ensure that this is then in the budget as a cost pressure in the relevant financial year. Flag this up with your Division's management team well in advance!

The template for business cases from one of our organizations has the following headings, which can be used as pointers for areas that you need to consider when putting a case together:

Outline business case

1. Objectives and identify benefit criteria
    i. Current situation
    ii. Supporting (or background) information
    iii. Benefit criteria
2. Strategic fit (local, regional, national)
3. Options considered and reason for preferred option
4. Benefits appraisal
    i. Patient experience
    ii. Strategic development
    iii. Financial contribution
5. Financial implications – identify and quantify revenue and capital costs
6. Impact of project – e.g. staff, facilities, capital, clinical support services
7. Implementation plan

If you are uncertain of the content – for example writing your first business case in a new organization, then try and show the first draft to a 'critical friend' either inside or outside the organization (though be certain to keep any Trust information confidential). It does not matter if they are not in palliative care; remember most of the people who will need to read this and be convinced by it, will not be. This will help you to avoid writing something incomprehensible or completely inadequate and having to recover from a 'bad start'.

Working within bureaucratic structures

NHS Trusts are bureaucratic structures and it is important that, however frustrating at time, you find ways of working within the system in order to be successful. When you understand your organisation and how it works, you will find that these systems can work for you and do not always need to be seen as against you. As Trusts have to be accountable to the SHA, Healthcare Commission, or Monitor, a certain degree of bureaucracy is inevitable. As a senior clinician, you also have bureaucratic obligations, for example to ensure that there are effective governance arrangements in place for your team or service (see Chapter 4 for more information).

It is important that you do not get too ground down or demoralized by seemingly slow progress or challenges in making real changes. You will need to play a long game and it may help to work with a colleague or mentor to review progress and set realistic goals. Getting team 'buy in' is also crucial, so that there is shared ownership of service developments (however small) and that you are able to devolve or delegate responsibility for some elements to other team members. Don't try to do everything yourself – it will become overwhelming and you will be at risk of becoming exhausted and demoralized.

Some key points that we have found useful are:

1. Make friends with your management team – they should be there to help and support you.

2. If you are not sure how to get some thing done, ask for help – from your colleagues, your clinical director, your manager – someone is likely to be able to help and support you.

3. Try to set realistic time lines.

4. Ensure that you involve your team in service developments so that they feel part of it and delegate responsibility for elements of implementation where you can – to share the load and also to ensure team involvement.

5. Book regular holidays and look after yourself – if you feel exhausted or demoralized, it may well be time to get some perspective.

6. Keep looking for opportunities with regard to strategy developments and funding that enable you to move your service forwards.

7. Never give up!

Outside of your organization

Cancer networks

In England and Wales there are 34 cancer networks, all of which have palliative care representative groups (or networks). The constituency and terms of reference of these groups may vary to an extent, but they are important in the strategic and collaborative development of palliative care services in localities and engagement is crucial. Most palliative care networks will have representation from their palliative care service providers, including NHS Trusts, usually from the lead clinician – in practice often a medical or nurse consultant or their representative. Attending these meetings and engagement with the palliative care network offers several advantages:

1. You get to meet other clinicians and key players locally, such as the commissioners. If you are new to a locality, this is absolutely key as success in your post will in part depend on forging successful working relationships with other service providers in your locality.

2. You get to understand how services fit together and are aware of local tensions and difficulties, which may be important to understand for your day to day practice.

3. You will start to understand the key issues that are affecting local services and the strategic drivers that are coming from the Department of Health which will also be debated and usually managed through the palliative care network – so you have an opportunity to understand key strategic issues and think through the implications for your Trust.

4. Network meetings are a good opportunity to meet up with colleagues and 'network' – both at the meeting and perhaps socially after, which is supportive and helpful!

5. The Network may also give you opportunities to identify funding to develop your services, for example via small amounts of 'slippage money' for specific projects (e.g. implementation of end of life care tools or for information technology). In previous years, larger sums of money have also been available for service developments and cancer/palliative care networks, in liaison with primary care trusts (PCTs), have coordinated the allocation – for example, the money allocated to specialist palliative and end-of-life care.

In most localities, in addition to the palliative care network, there will also be more local groups, usually operating within PCT boundaries, either as part of cancer locality groups or as separate palliative care locality groups. There are geographical differences, but you may find that more 'work' is done through the locality groups whereas the network groups are more strategic – so the crucial thing is to understand *how things work in your area* and to target the key meetings that you need to be involved in. Changing services is often linked to a specific person or small number of people who drive projects; in practice, they do more than attend meetings and also undertake work between meetings and do not leave issues alone. You will need to convince these 'doers' about the rightness of your policies or strategic changes.

In addition to the PCT cancer or palliative care groups, most palliative care networks will have a range of subgroups that you may wish to get involved in, depending on your interest and expertise. Alternatively, you may identify other members of your team who *may wish* to get involved in such groups, in order to develop their skills, thereby sharing the meeting load around. If different team members are attending different meetings, then it is also vital to have feedback mechanisms within your service so that you are all kept up to date and have an opportunity to input into local developments.

Cancer networks will also have a range of site-specific tumour working groups and a research network group, all of whom should have palliative care representation. This is usually coordinated through the network palliative care group – so if you have a particular interest in attending one of these groups with a view to developing services or furthering research interests, attendance as the palliative care representative is a good way in.

The risk with the cancer network and the myriad of sub-groups is that you could spend your life attending meetings rather than developing and delivering a clinical service back at base. Working as a senior member of a multi-professional team, it should be possible to identify other senior people with whom you can share out meeting attendance, so that key meetings are covered and your service is adequately represented. Targeting key meetings is crucial and is an excellent way of keeping informed of regional and national initiatives that may take on direct relevance for your service (e.g. Picture for Health in London and the Darzi report nationally). Make sure whoever goes to the meeting is adequately prepared and able to contribute in a positive way.

Regional and national initiatives

As you become more experienced, more confident and start to develop key areas of interest, you may wish to explore the opportunities for being involved in national groups. Examples include:

1. National Council for Palliative Care policy groups (see *http://www.ncpc.org. uk/policy_unit/policy_groups.htm*) – these groups usually require you to be something of an 'expert' in the area
2. NCRI palliative care studies subgroups – see Chapter 9 for further detail on research groups

3. APM groups (*http://www.palliative-medicine.org/*), e.g. professional development committee, science committee

4. Working groups related to regional or national initiatives, e.g. end-of-life care

Money, money, money

Financing palliative care services is a complex issue and although salaries and terms and conditions of service are to an extent protected within NHS services, you will soon start wanting to explore ways in which you can finance equipment, other resources, and service developments.

A detailed discussion of the complexities of NHS funding are beyond the remit of this book, however, most hospital services are linked to funding agreements or payment by results, whereby funding is linked to clinical activity. At present NHS hospital palliative care services do not have a tariff (anticipated as part of HRG4 in 2009/10[4]), so palliative care services in hospitals currently are effectively funded by 'top slicing' from the tariffs attached to other clinical services and activities. In the current economic climate, the lack of a defined income related to activity can be seen as a potential risk, unless you can be certain that you are seen as central to patient care by the most powerful members of the hospital team.

Developing services therefore relies on identifying local and national resources for securing additional funding.

Local resources

Most Trusts have their own charity and fundraising departments; the size of these charities varies and in our experience some hospital charities will pump-prime clinical or research posts but some will not. Where funding for posts is not available, however, Trust charities may be able to be utilized to purchase equipment, e.g. syringe drivers. Trust fundraising teams tend to focus on large projects, often involving capital re-building, but there may be opportunities for you to piggy-back onto an existing of proposed large project to obtain further resource for your service.

In 2010–11 it is proposed that payment by results (PbR) will be extended under Health Resource Group (HRG) 4 to include specialist palliative care services. HRG4 addresses clinical areas that have traditionally used departmental data recording systems that might not be linked to patient administration systems (PAS). In order for your Trust to receive income related to

---

[4] *http://www.ic.nhs.uk/casemix/prepare.*

palliative care activity, the Trust needs to set up processes and systems to ensure that data with respect to palliative care episodes is made available for coding. Clinical coders are unlikely to be familiar with the data collected on palliative care databases and will not have experience of applying Office of Population Censuses and Surveys (OPCS) coding to this data. You will therefore need to work with your management team and the Trust clinical coding team to identify a system so that palliative care activity can be coded. Once income can be identified relating to palliative care, there is the potential for identifying local funding for service development.

It is also possible to obtain additional resources through your Trust to develop services, but with the current financial constraints this very much depends on the financial security of the Trust and the impact of any likely service reorganisations. In practice, Foundation Trusts have the ability to keep and re-invest any surpluses, so this may enable opportunities for investment. Any successful bid for funds will depend, however, on a successful business case and it is therefore crucial that you are able to evidence benefit for the organization as a result of any new investment. In our experience, working collaboratively with your organization's management is absolutely crucial in taking successful business cases and service development ideas forward.

National resources

National charities, e.g. Marie Curie, Macmillan Cancer Support and non-cancer charities, such as the British Lung Foundation, British Heart Foundation, Multiple Sclerosis Society, and the Motor Neurone Disease Association, all have track records for funding (in practice usually pump-priming) posts. The criteria for applications will vary year on year, so it is most useful to make contact with the local service development manager for the charity to discuss any proposals you have in order to see whether this is something that they will then consider funding.

National initiatives, e.g. £50 million for palliative care in 2003 to 2006 and the recent end-of-life care funding provide further opportunities for exploring opportunities for investing in your service – for equipment, teaching and training resources, and potentially for staff. Allocation of these resources is usually co-ordinated through network palliative care groups, so engagement in these groups is crucial. It is anticipated that the £286 million funding accompanying the 2008 End of Life Care Strategy[5] will be distributed via primary care trusts, but no detailed information is currently available regarding this; however,

---

[5] *http://www.dh.gov.uk/en/Publicationsandstatistics/Publications/Publications-PolicyAndGuidance/DH_086277.*

it is likely that much of this funding will be to support the development of generalist services to support more people dying at home and in workforce development.

Developing your management skills

In order to function successfully as a consultant or other senior clinician, it is important to think about developing your management skills. Many specialist registrars will have done management courses as part of their training and some nurse specialists will have had the opportunity to develop management and/or leadership skills. Whilst there is no replacement for rolling up your sleeves and getting stuck in – and, to an extent, learning as you go, it is also useful to explore opportunities to underpin your increasing experience with some theory.

Many hospital Trusts run management development courses for new (medical) consultants – if available, these are well worth attending, not only for the theory but also as an opportunity to meet colleagues, to network, and to learn by shared experiences.

Regional and national organizations also run successful management courses, for example the King's Fund (you can view the relevant courses available at *http://www.kingsfund.org.uk/leadership/open_programmes.html*). Your local postgraduate medical centre or director of nursing may be a useful resource in researching what is available, what your Trust will fund, and what would be best for you. Developing your management skills are also something that can be discussed as part of the annual appraisal process and contribute to your personal development plan.

The Royal College of Physicians is running a leadership course which can lead to an MSc. If you are just starting: think about how you can best get the management skills to help you achieve your goals and be happy in your work. Bureaucracy and management are inescapable facts of life.

Summary

A detailed understanding of the structure of the wider NHS as well as the way *your* hospital, locality, and network function operates at a strategic level is essential if you are going to develop your service effectively.

Chapter 7

Education in the acute hospital

There is no single way of delivering education in acute Trusts. It is essential for success that education is tailored to your Trust and the people who work there: the 'who, why, where, what and how' will follow this. You always have limited time, you are not an education service and do not have the resources of one, so target it to unmet needs that you have identified and can meet.

Many groups (such as undergraduate nurses, doctors, and therapists) will already have structured education programmes, following nationally-defined curricula with which you can work. It is likely that the academic staff responsible for these courses will be knocking on your door, as palliative care is increasingly recognized as a generic skill which needs to be an intrinsic part of undergraduate courses.

A pre-existing structure and recognized need for palliative care education will also operate for some postgraduate courses such as those for FY1 and 2 doctors; detailed discussion of the content for these groups will not be covered in this chapter (recommended reading is given at the end) but an outline of some ideas to help you get involved in such work in the most effective way.

It is important to remember the time necessary to plan and deliver any education: universities, schools, and other centres of education invest huge amounts of time and employ dedicated administrative staff when preparing course materials and planning the ways that they will educate students under their care. Delivering education to larger number of people at once is more efficient (although not always most effective, depending on the topic). You will not have the time and support for comprehensive education programmes or full-time educationalists but consider:

1. Pooling your resources: your network will have a strategy for education (or be working on one) join in and conduct joint teaching sessions; you may have a neighbouring hospice with whom you can work collaboratively planning some of your education with them so that you do not duplicate and can teach on each other courses. Bringing together people who would usually separately attend community and acute trust courses may also have additional benefits such as improving communication.

2. Giving participants something they can use in their professional portfolios: everyone has to justify and cost any time spent on education. Get your courses accredited for continuing professional development (CPD) points, where possible, by the relevant professional colleges or groups. Issue a certificate of attendance for participants whether it is accredited or not.

3. Finding out what your Trust needs: palliative care can teach many skills that may be of use to groups who are rarely targeted for education (e.g. communication skills for clinic receptionists). You would need to organize and teach this with their 'line managers' so that skills they consider relevant are taught as well as the ones you have observed to be needed. You would gain influence and possibly time and money to prepare course materials if you can do this.

4. Using professionally prepared or bespoke teaching material where available: you will usually have to pay someone for this (after all they have spent money and time preparing them), but it may be a good investment. The time you invest in customizing them for your setting will be less than the time they put in preparing the originals.

5. Pooling slides and teaching materials within a team so that people do not have to endlessly prepare very similar material; individuals will probably want to 'customize' material for their own presentations but it will save some preparation time.

6. There will be learning and training department for Trust staff to deliver Trust initiatives (e.g. management or diversity training). You may be able to link up with them to save valuable time and resources or to carry out a 'needs assessment' within your hospital.

Always find out where you can team up with Trust or academic initiatives as pushing through training programmes solely in the capacity as a palliative care team is hard work; you may put in much effort and time for limited attendance and impact.

Delivering education

Delivering education can be considered using the headings: Who? How? Why? What? When? Where?

Who to teach?

This could be answered in one word: 'everyone', but that would not be helpful as palliative care teams are ostensibly employed for a mainly clinical remit and you will not have the time in your job plans (or perhaps the training) to accomplish initiatives of significant scope unaided by Trust or Directorate support.

Palliative care teams will almost certainly, almost automatically, be involved in teaching doctors and nurses and this teaching will be ward based and in pre-existing education programmes: but unless you have an allied health professional (AHP) in your team, it is easy to overlook this group. Do make contact with the managers of physiotherapy, speech therapy, occupational therapy, and dietetics to see how best to deliver education to these groups. Don't forget pharmacy as well. Remember that turnover in junior and training grades in Trusts will be rapid, so any education will certainly need to be part of a rolling programme, preferably integrated into existing supported departmental training programmes.

It is always a moot point whether to educate the clinical managers of a department or the staff in lower bands or training grades. The former may set the tone and culture for the ward or department but will not have a much direct clinical contact. Those in lower training bands will move on (often to other hospitals), but you may make a bigger individual impact. This will be a decision for your team in your Trust, but needs consideration and your decision and strategy intermittently reviewed for its effectiveness.

There are certain staff who are often overlooked, for example:

1. Health Care Assistants

2. Non-clinical (e.g. clerical) staff

Their education may be confined to mandatory training such as fire lectures and 'moving and handling', but they are rarely offered the opportunity to develop in other ways. We would argue that improving the communication skills of these staff should be a priority. They are often the first people to have contact with a patient when they arrive at hospital, and equipping them with the knowledge and skills of how to interact with patients, can go a long way to ensuring that the patient experience is positive from the outset.

Many clinical and non-clinical disciplines within the hospital are already linked into regular education programmes within their own specific areas. Approach departmental heads who will often be delighted to give Palliative Care the opportunity to speak at one of their teaching sessions: this is a good chance to highlight the remit of the Palliative Care team and make clear how get in touch.

Specific groups: undergraduate medical students

Many acute hospital Trusts, if not designated teaching hospitals, are now affiliated to medical schools, which gives the opportunity to be involved in medical student teaching. This can be extremely rewarding, especially where basic palliative care skills are key to the competencies expected of a Foundation year 1 doctor (that is, those doctors straight out of medical school).

Nowadays, most medical schools have palliative medicine teaching within their curriculum; although how this is delivered (e.g. an integrated programme over the whole course, a block of designated teaching, perhaps linked to oncology, or a mix of both, varies enormously between schools). If it does not appear that there is much teaching that may be an opportunity to get involved – but this is likely to take considerable time and effort, so be prepared! At one of our medical schools, we deliver a now well-established integrated programme over the 5-year course. However, 10 years ago the teaching was minimal and very fragmented. In developing the teaching programme we mapped the Association of Palliative Medicine palliative medicine curriculum onto the medical school's curriculum, met key players to understand how the curriculum was evolving (with the introduction of a new curriculum and medical school merger), and then went about identifying where we and how we could deliver teaching to meet the need. Getting started required enthusiasm, energy, and commitment from a group of consultants, with several of us attending curriculum meetings over many months (and years) in order to achieve our objectives. Since then, clear teaching objectives, a mix of teaching methods, and regular evaluation and course revision have all helped us deliver a teaching programme that is respected and well evaluated – with which in turn, it is rewarding to be involved.

If there is an established undergraduate palliative care teaching programme in place at your local medical school, in the first instance it is useful to make contact with the palliative care teaching lead in order to understand what teaching is delivered, where it is delivered, and by whom. It may be that they are looking for more teachers to be involved in clinical teaching to facilitate small group teaching, to help support seminar and symposia programmes, and to get involved in examining students. If medical students undertake placements at your hospital, then there may be opportunities to set up clinical teaching and you may be approached by colleagues asking you to get involved. In our experience, all such opportunities should be greeted with enthusiasm and taken, as there is often considerable competition for teaching time within the curriculum. It is helpful, however, to keep the link with the medical school teaching lead so that the teaching that you deliver is broadly in line with the overall palliative medicine undergraduate curriculum and that all teaching is integrated. Students get bored and vocal if there is obvious overlap and repetition (although the latter, cleverly disguised, is necessary if key information is to be remembered).

We all work at institutions where palliative care teaching is greatly supported by our medical schools and where integrated curricula are the norm, but that does not mean medical students will always give palliative care a priority and most important way of getting palliative care prioritized by students is to ensure that it is *examined*. Therefore, try and get involved, or ensure that someone from the region is involved (you cannot do everything) in setting questions and do take any opportunities to be examiners for Objective Structured Clinical Examinations (OSCEs).

Being involved in the medical school has other benefits:

1. You will keep up your skills and may get some further training in teaching and examining.

2. You will meet other specialists and there is little time available now for meeting other clinicians in the working day except when talking about a specific patient: you may convert them to the value of palliative care or at least give them an insight into the specialty.

3. You may make a friend outside your immediate department (see Chapter 10).

4. You may develop an interest which will take you beyond palliative care alone (see Chapter 10).

5. You will reflect on your own practice.

6. You will get peer review at the examiners' meetings both on clinical practice and on your own teaching skills.

How to teach

Once a decision has been made regarding whom to teach, the next problem to be tackled is *how*. Not everyone learns well in a classroom environment. Education theories suggest that using a mix of teaching styles is most effective and should be considered when delivering any formal education. A detailed discussion on teaching and learning styles is outside of the remit of this book, but some resources are listed at the end of this chapter to help you.

In practice, however, much of the education delivered by hospital palliative care teams is not formal – for example, learning through shadowing or infor-mal ward-based teaching.

Informal education

Even though it is very labour intensive, the one-to-one approach is often use-ful, giving an opportunity for role modelling. This involves a shadowing opportunity, where a member of staff goes about their normal work but has another person watching how they undertake it. There is plenty of scope for immediate discussion, of the problems of the patients being seen and a chance to give a detailed account of how palliative care management decisions are reached. Many teams have to limit the number of team 'shadowing' experience they are prepared to offer because

1. They are hard on the clinician being shadowed because of the scrutiny.

2. They are time-consuming.

3. The learner may visit on a day when there are too few patients and therefore little of interest or conversely, when the team feel too busy to be able to talk things through in detail.

4. Being shadowed is tiring because of the need to explain everything in depth.

5. It is also very dependant on what turns up during that morning's work.

There are less easily measured benefits to being shadowed:

1. You will enhance or develop relationships with members of other departments who know little about your work or who are new to the Trust and may be able to support you in unforeseen ways.

2. The scrutiny encourages you to reflect on your practice.

3. Sometimes the person who accompanies you has some useful clinical knowledge or contact or ideas to improve the care of the patients you see that morning and changes your practice in the future.

Teaching those who consult the team

Informal opportunities commonly arise in day-to-day practice. There may be opportunities at the bedside for teaching student nurses or junior doctors when you have asked to see a patient. This is particularly useful for highlighting how to handle a difficult symptom or situation, however, there is no way to evaluate the learning and it would be rare to have written information to give out for reinforcement. Encouraging visiting or junior clinicians to attend at clinics, with the patient's permission, also gives the opportunity for a detailed discussion on palliative care problems. This is usually a quieter environment than the ward allowing a more focussed discussion. Outpatients often have a large number of complex problems and as they tend to be fitter than inpatients, there is scope for a wider range of interventions.

Educational opportunities arise everywhere and do not necessarily have to be formal or within a structured framework. Bedside and 'on the job' education often has more impact. A 'case in point' can be discussed with the patients' permission and opportunity for discussion including the patient is frequently valuable. Striving for user involvement is one of the key principles of palliative care as it enables the patient voice to be heard in the decision-making process.

Sentinel event or significant event analysis

It is important and often powerful to learn from events when they have not gone according to plan or as hoped. Taking the opportunity to scrutinize with the whole team and without recrimination or blame, what could have been done better or alternatively how the best was done even though the results were disappointing gives the chance for concerns to be aired within a safe environment. This type of significant event analysis often forges better relationships within teams and fosters a culture of learning and enquiry.

Training needs may also be identified by feedback from adverse incidents and complaints on certain wards or for certain teams; those relevant to palliative care often relate to the administration or delivery of analgesics and other symptom control medication and communication. Many arise from end-of-life care, which is perceived by relatives or friends to have been sub-standard.

A more individual opportunity for learning can be encouraged by utilizing reflective diaries, where it is possible to examine personal actions and examine whether we could or would do something differently given a similar situation.

Both these different learning tools can also give teams the chance to celebrate successes. Reflection does not necessarily have to be negative!

Case study: Teaching communication skills to oncology junior doctors

One of us ran a project with oncology trainees where they had a palliative care mentor (from the medical team) and used a tutorial system centred on patients on the ward. It was very time consuming, the impact was uncertain, and was discontinued for this reason.

A more successful initiative was set up by a palliative medicine consultant but run by the communication skills unit. Once a month the oncology trainees were asked to bring their lunch to one of the outpatients rooms; here they worked with a 'simulated patient' (actor) and senior communication skills tutor. They were encouraged to use their own experiences with patients and colleagues on the ward and to replay those they had found difficult, emotionally taxing or where they wished they had 'said something else'. The money for the actor came from the oncology charitable funds and the training was very highly evaluated by the trainees. Other sessions were run in the regular oncology 'audit academic meeting' for registrars and consultants.

Informal education, participating in other teams academic meetings, and 'on the job' teaching are the methods that are the most likely to reach consultants and specialist nurses in other disciplines who will not use their study leave budgets of time or money to go on specialist palliative care courses.

Reaching other specialists with advanced education is one of the most difficult issues for specialist palliative care teams: ensure you take every chance you can get but do not be disheartened if progress seems to be slow. You may have to try (and fail sometimes) using different methods to reach different teams.

Formal education

The training of nurses, doctors, and allied health professionals (AHPs) is curriculum based. Where possible, linking in with higher educational institutions (HEIs) potentially enables involvement at the curriculum planning stage and subsequent participation in courses; it is an effective and efficient way to teach a number of staff at the same time. Most HEI tutors welcome this input and are pleased to have representation from clinical staff at their planning meetings. Many HEIs will give honorary lecturer status to those who have a set amount of input into their courses, which is always useful on the CV! Some institutions will pay the teacher or their department.

Preparing for teaching

Never underestimate the time it takes to prepare a teaching session and do not forget to update your presentations periodically (for similar audiences) and rework them for every outside meeting that you go to. All this takes time and it is easy to say 'yes' to something 3 months ahead and then be unable to put in the necessary time to prepare a good presentation. This doesn't mean turn everything down unless you can do it perfectly, but it does mean:

1. Be realistic about what you can take on.
2. Do not take on completely new subjects too often.
3. Work with another team member on tricky occasions or difficult subjects or seminars and workshops.
4. Do prepare carefully for events which require spontaneity (sic), e.g. workshops.
5. Put update 'deadlines' on footers of your handouts.
6. Do not work on automatic pilot: jut because a session was done as a lecture last time does not mean it should be done this way again, perhaps a workshop would be better.
7. Do start to think about e-learning.

Remember you do need to teach in lots of different ways and formats if you are to change the culture of the acute Trust.

Structuring teaching sessions

All formal teaching should ideally be delivered as part of a structured programme, informed by a training needs analysis. Such teaching may take the form of study days or half days; regular seminar slots as part of ward-based teaching programmes; a rolling programme of teaching informed by competencies, e.g. syringe driver teaching; or part of undergraduate or postgraduate programmes.

No matter what method is employed to deliver the training, *learning aims and objectives* for the session should be set at the outset, and revisited at the end to ensure they have been met. In a larger meeting this may be something you decide and publicize beforehand (useful to delegates to know if it will meet their needs). *Knowing your audience* is also crucial: it is especially helpful to clarify the level at which the training is pitched.

For example a seminar entitled 'The Management of Bowel Obstruction' could be aimed at

1. The gynaeoncology MDT (including palliative care)
2. The colorectal MDT
3. The ward staff on the gynaeoncology ward
4. The ward staff on a surgical ward
5. The ward staff on an oncology ward
6. SpRs in palliative care in the region
7. SpRs in obs and gynae in the region
8. Surgical SpRs in the region
9. Oncology SpRs in the region
10. National conferences for palliative care clinicians
11. National conferences for palliative care medics, or nurses
12. Undergraduates in medicine or nursing
13. Pharmacists
14. Dieticians
15. Radiographers

All these audiences will have overlapping and individual needs which must be identified and met if the seminar is to be useful for the individuals concerned. When you publicize it, make sure you make it clear who the seminar is primarily aimed at, how you are going to teach it, and the learning objectives.

With small groups and more informal teaching the learning objectives can be discussed with the group at the beginning of the session, displayed on a flipchart, and returned to intermittently during the session.

It is also important to consider how to meet people's learning needs by *incorporating different learning styles* into the teaching programme. In our experience, in any teaching session, however short, a mix of teaching styles is key to engage as many of the audience as possible, as people learn in different ways. Some people learn better with a didactic 'chalk and talk' session. Others find this very off-putting. More useful may be the workshop, which are participative and where staff learn in small groups and undertake problem-solving sessions. However, this type of teaching will require skilled facilitation, therefore more staff will be required to deliver the session. Often a mixture of both types of teaching will benefit the majority. Examples of different teaching methods that can be incorporated into a teaching session are given below:

1. Start the session with a buzz group (small groups of two to three, talking about a key issue, potentially involving feedback to the teaching lead): this can wake everyone up!

2. Small group discussions, perhaps around a clinical case or problem, potentially including feedback to the wider group

3. Using video material to illustrate clinical points

4. Using debate to cover the pros and cons of a specific issue

Linking case examples to teaching that illustrate common problems in a non-judgemental way can also help to bring learning alive and make it clinically relevant.

Even apparently unstructured teaching sessions need extensive planning: the first time a new session is carried out, the preparation time will be at least double the time needed for the session itself.

Once given, it is good practice to review even well-evaluated sessions at least annually and to make sure that they have not been superseded by teaching given in other session that the students receive.

Case study: Death and Dying course

A 'Death and Dying' course was started in conjunction with the communications skills department and a number of other supportive clinicians (including pathology, A&E, oncology) and other disciplines involved with patients, families, or their issues (e.g. chaplaincy, coroner's officer) around the time of death. When the course was begun, there was very little in the medical school curriculum on palliative care: during the next 7 years the medical school paid more attention to this subject and the palliative care lectures on the course, as well the bereavement sessions were changed – the time could be used to consider more advanced issues in this subject area. As well as being a successful module for the medical students, it was a valuable opportunity for palliative care to be involved in other departments who rarely met them.

It is useful to go through a *checklist* for formal all day or half-day teaching sessions, including national events:

1. Have you decided on objectives for the day?

2. Have you decided who is best to teach the required sessions?

3. If they are ones your team have taught before, remember to look at the teaching materials in good time: they may well need updating.

4. If using 'inside' speakers, have you worked out how to keep the clinical service going that day (see Box 7.2)?

5. If using 'outside' speakers, have you worked out the costs (travelling expenses and accommodation will add significantly to your bill)?

6. Have you organized enough advertising and publicity targeted to the delegates you want to attract?

7. Have you organized refreshments and a way of only ordering the amount you need?

8. What will be the cancellation costs for any venue you have paid for?

9. Have you organized hand-outs or other supporting materials?

10. Have you organized A-V support for the day? (If you need lap-tops/projectors, it will be expensive if you do not bring your own.)

11. Do you have enough rooms for break-out sessions? .

12. Have you got an easy booking system?

13. Have you organized troubleshooter on the day (not involved in the teaching and able to sort out problems)?

14. Have you organized a time to go through the evaluations and debrief with the team afterwards (not necessarily that day)?

15. Have you organized expenses claims for your speakers

We think that it is usually preferable to keep training and education planning as simple as possible and avoid the use of paid venues (however sumptuous) unless it is unavoidable. Many Trusts are not prepared to pay for outside education for their staff, particularly outside the region, so even the best training days or conferences (see later) may be poorly attended; it is certainly not a good way of making money for the team. On the other hand, organizing your own conference and bringing in outside speakers and delegates is a cost-effective way of bringing education to your region and may 'break even' if carried out in partnership with other palliative care teams or hospices. More on national days is found later on p. 111.

Sponsorship for teaching

This is a complex and contentious issue. Many clinicians are concerned about taking money from drug companies as they feel a pressure of reciprocity even if this is not discussed. Many Trusts no longer permit their staff to obtain sponsorship from pharmaceutical companies, which in turn are bound by the Association of Pharmaceutical Industry guidelines. Recent guidance suggests that the practice of a system of continuing education funded by an industry with a vested interest in promoting its products is no longer acceptable, but in practice limited central funding means that pharmaceutical support is still often required to enable the delivery of formal education, ranging from giving lunch to attract ward staff to learner-centred practices (LCP) teaching sessions and to national conferences with subsidised places for Trust staff, keeping the costs manageable.

Case study: Planning multi-professional palliative care teaching

An innovative approach that we have adopted is an Integrated Teaching Programme. This is planned and delivered by the multi-professional palliative care team from across the area.

All team members have made a commitment to deliver sessions and the dates are booked a year in advance. This enables the teaching to become a part of the working week, and because all members of the wider team are enlisted, this approach reduces the burden from the few and spreads it across the wider team. It also gives the opportunity for different perspectives to be highlighted during training, as the problems which arise in the hospital will undoubtedly be very different in the palliative care team.

Length of formal sessions

It is moot point whether teaching is best given as half or whole day sessions. Most staff seems to find it easier to be released for a whole rather than a half day.

Other considerations under 'when' and 'where'

Although ward teaching at lunchtime or during the working day seems an attractive way of reaching clinicians where they are and providing education for those who would not attend more formal specialist palliative care training, it is possible for you to spend a lot of time preparing and organizing such sessions to find that on the day only one or two people can be spared to attend and even then, they may be interrupted or unable to concentrate because of shortages on the ward. Most of these sessions have improved attendance if lunch is provided, but many people will leave early and you may feel let down.

This happens even with quite extensive preparation beforehand and can be demoralizing. This is always a tactic worth considering but not worth pursuing when it is not working as it is a common experience at acute hospitals. It is often more successful to ensure that you have a teaching opportunity on a team or department study day when the education will be supported by that group. Such days are commonly multi-disciplinary and whilst this may give some difficulties in structuring the teaching so that everyone gets something from it, there is the bonus of reaching 'hard to meet' groups.

This only underlines the importance of not having fixed ideas of about how and where to educate but tailoring it to the team you want to introduce to your service or to the ideas of palliative care.

Here are some other ideas:

1. Drop in sessions with 1/2 hour talks on specific subjects and lunch available for anyone in the hospital, advertised through the hospital internet communication system. These can be run with other teams such as acute and chronic pain.

2. Drop by sessions with palliative care manning a exhibition or with written materials to offer to patients and staff alike in a very public part of the hospital.

3. Running seminars or teaching sessions with the postgraduate centre for GPs and other members of the primary care team. These will often by well advertised by them and already a 'recognized' event on the calendar.

4. Running short items in your hospital paper or newsletter: always use the appointment of a new member of staff as an opportunity to have a short article or paragraph introducing them to the wider hospital community. It reminds everyone of the existence and function of the team.

5. Taking part in the hospital annual public meeting or open day.

6. Making sure that any posters that you have prepared for academic meetings are displayed at any other exhibition or demonstration that departments of the trust are organizing.

If training is more formal and is to be delivered within a classroom, the first difficulty is usually finding accommodation. Most on-site education centres will have IT support, therefore standard training equipment should be available which should include as a minimum:

1. Computers

2. PowerPoint projectors

3. Whiteboards (electronic in some cases)

4. Overhead projectors

5. Flipcharts

For Trust staff most education centres room-bookings will be free of charge. If accommodation cannot be found on site, there may be major difficulty in running the course and in the extra travelling time for staff. The cost of venues is a major factor when considering training, especially when most Trusts have reduced the amount of money available to deliver or receive education.

Evaluation of teaching

As important as well planned and delivered teaching is the evaluation of a session. This usually involves the completion of a simple form combining predetermined questions, often with a scoring range to choose, and an opportunity for individual responses in free text. Other, less commonly used methods of evaluation can be helpful, e.g. responses to a quiz at the end of the session testing knowledge gained during it, or simple traffic lights approaches such as asking attendees to record what they would like the teachers to:

1. Stop doing ……. (red)

2. Do more of …… (green)

3. Do in a different way …..(amber)

Many people attending educational events find evaluation forms hard to fill in. It can be helpful to hand them out at the beginning of the session and have each topic evaluated as it is delivered. That way there is more likelihood that the actual feedback delivered will be relevant and not just a distant memory! At all-day events it is usual for at least some of the audience to leave early and there are nearly always late-comers; the numbers of evaluations can be disappointing and if you are really keen to have it, for a new course perhaps, evaluation may need to be planned (even if not listed) before the last session or as part of the last session.

However, this form of face-to-face feedback may also be influenced by being so closely linked to the teachers that evidence suggests that evaluation after an event (on paper or online) may be more objective. It is also useful to consider further evaluation some weeks or months after an event to consider whether and improvements in knowledge, skills, or attitudes have been maintained. These last options are rarely done for practical reasons but there is now a considerable body of medical and nursing education literature so consulting experts or looking up the evidence on evaluation could bear fruit.

Once the evaluations have been received, take time to look at them closely. Positive feedback is always good; however, feedback that may initially appear to be critical is also very helpful. Acting on feedback can make the difference between having well attended and poorly attended sessions.

Giving certificates of attendance is a good idea even if the session has not been validated or accredited. The addition of certificates for portfolios is now essential as proof of ongoing professional development.

To link or not to link?

Link nurses? Love them or hate them? It has to be said that in some areas having a dedicated nurse to act as the link for a particular subject works incredibly well. In others it is an unmitigated disaster. Difficulties may arise if there are several 'link' nurses on each ward as it may be that the responsibility for that particular area of practice then rests with them. They will probably be extremely efficient and hopefully have good up-to-date knowledge for their area of expertise, but may not have the time or opportunity to cascade the knowledge to others. There may be a tendency from other staff to refer patients directly to the link nurse rather than enhance their own skills and knowledge. Consequently when the link nurse is on annual leave, sick leave or moved to another clinical area the knowledge base is lost.

In areas where link nurses work well, there is often a cascade mechanism in place where the knowledge is shared. This could take the form of a brief update on symptom management or innovative practice. This works particularly well when integrated into handover time, as the maximum number of staff can benefit. Having a resource folder on the ward also works, although this will need to be updated regularly. Reporting back from conferences or study days is also a good way to cascade information to a number of staff where there are limited resources for attendance at such events.

Clinical skills can be enhanced by the shadowing process where a member of staff learns skills directly form the link nurse. Examples where this could be used are in areas such as setting up a syringe driver or observing an interaction to enhance communication skills.

The quality of the link nurse's work very much depends on

1. Whether he/she was designated or volunteered

2. Whether they have the remotest interest in the subject

3. Whether they are team players or see this as a covert opportunity to develop their own skills and knowledge with the minimum of effort

4. Whether the role is supported by an educational framework or is it just a tick box exercise

5. How many other link roles that particularly nurse or ward is involved with already? Recent work at one of our Trusts revealed that some individuals were carrying as many as 11 link specialities and there were over 25 on the wards.

We have known both scenarios in our careers and it very much depends on the individual establishments and the nurses themselves whether the link nurse role is effective or not. Suffice for it to say for the scheme to work the link nurse has to be capable of cascading and sharing the skills and knowledge she has learnt and has a commitment to the development of other staff.

National study days

Most one day national days are now put on by the teams linked with journals or well-established organizations. The effort that is required to put on a national study day is unbelievable. Planning for these days starts at least 12 months before the actual event and requires a dedicated team for Project Management. The following are some of the many things that will need to be considered:

1. Subject matter

2. Target audience

3. Venue

4. Didactic sessions or to include workshops

5. Cost for delegates

6. Sponsorship of the event

7. Catering

8. Speakers

9. Publicity and advertising

10. Timing of event

11. IT support

12. Database of delegates

13. Mail shots to delegates

14. Handling monies

15. Cut-off date for cancellation

16. Venue costs for cancellation

Planning such an event is very time consuming and not to be undertaken lightly. The timing of the event is crucial and the organizing team need to be aware of other events, which are taking place around the same time, as these will be direct competitors for the target audience. Also including 'hot topics' is often a risky plan. What may be 'hot' at the time of planning could be very old news at the time of delivery.

All these things aside it is a very satisfying process to see long thought-out plans come to fruition. Equally it can be soul destroying to have gone down the route of staging such an event and having to cancel at the eleventh hour because of lack of delegates.

Whether trying to support a national day or undertaking local training, it's often worth linking in with Cancer Networks to find out whether they have any additional money that can support such events.

Almost every Trust in the UK has had to make savings and one of the first things to be depleted was the training and education budget. Opportunities may arise when providing training linked to local initiative such as communication skills training and training on the end–of-life tools. Because these are national initiatives, it may be possible to link with a national training plan. This has dual benefits of the funding being obtained from the Government on your behalf and by having a captive audience ready and waiting for you! This can also mean that participants start with a feeling of not 'being there by choice' which you may need to overcome at the beginning of the day.

Do not forget to thank your speakers afterwards and give them some feedback on their presentation. Have a simple way for them to claim any expenses due.

Postgraduate studies for you

For many nurses and junior doctors the first degree is just the start of a period of lifelong learning. More and more clinical staff are engaging in postgraduate studies either to Certificate, Diploma, Masters, or Doctoral level. However, difficulties arise in obtaining time to study and funding for courses.

Decisions will need to be made how to study. There are opportunities to study at postgraduate level with courses offering opportunities for full time, part time, or distance learning. Equally there are choices between taught courses and research degrees, with doctoral studies now also offering a professional PhD, where the qualification is undertaken as part of the normal working day, with the choice of subject being part of the normal working environment of the student.

Postgraduate qualifications now have much more of a focus on assignments, essays, case studies, and projects. There is far less emphasis on formal examinations.

Another relatively new innovation is the Credit Accumulation Modular Scheme (CAMS) for some postgraduate courses. This may be available on part-time courses where the study is on a self-contained modular basis. Credits are awarded for each module and accumulated towards the final award. By accumulating credits in this way it is possible to change routes of transfer between higher education establishments whilst still undertaking further study.

Obtaining funding for courses will need to be considered. Unfortunately education does not come cheap and the as a student you may well be expected to at least secure some monies yourself. Before embarking on the route of student and bank loans or even adding to credit card debt, it is worth trying to obtain some funding from educational establishments. Some universities offer postgraduate bursaries, so in the first instance ask the questions of the higher education institution (HEI) where you would like to study.

Alternative sources of funding are available. Macmillan Cancer Support may be able to provide a grant for Macmillan-funded staff. Equally NHS student bursaries are available. If all else fails spending some time trawling through Google websites may throw up some funding sources. Some areas worth investigating are *www.mrc.ac.uk* (Medical Research Council), *www.educationuk. org/scholarships*, and *www.npc.org.uk* who have a good postgraduate funding guide available. Of course, these are only a few of many available and it is worth a good internet search to locate others.

Case study: Time for research

Neil was 5 years into his consultant job. He had always liked research and had done an MSc during his SpR training – that all seemed a very long time ago now. He then saw an advert for a scheme, funded by CeCo that gave clinicians 3 months off from clinical duties to complete a grant application. He applied and was successful, and an SpR from the rotation 'acted up' while he was off working with the other consultant in the department. The grant application was successful and so he obtained funding to carry out a clinical research project with data collection and writing up mainly carried out by a research associate. The department has continued research ever since.

Summary

Education is a core activity of any palliative care service. You will find there is much enthusiasm for the idea of education but often practical difficulties in finding ways to fit it into the hospital routine. You will need to be creative and part of the hospital mainstream to achieve your goals having a clear understanding of the needs of the staff working in your hospital. Do not assume that everyone in your team can teach; investment in training around teaching and presentation skills is money well spent. Collaboration enables you to avoid duplication, builds relationships with another departments, and pools resources.

Learning style resources

1. *http://www.mcpcil.org.uk/education/study_programmes/training_the_teachers* and *http://www.mcpcil.org.uk/education/study_programmes/training_the_trainers*
2. *http://www.learningfromexperience.com/*
3. *http://www.learning-theories.com/*

Chapter 8

Training issues in palliative medicine

Medical training

Palliative Medicine has been a recognized medical specialty in the UK since 1987, with a well-established pathway for postgraduate training. In order to understand this, it is important to have some knowledge of the structure of training and the various bodies that oversee it. This is set out below: the controversies attached to the various recent changes are not discussed.

Postgraduate training in the UK

Modernising Medical Careers (MMC) aimed to improve patient care by delivering an up-to-date and focused career structure for doctors. However, following on from the significant issues following implementation of MMC in the UK in 2007, the Government commissioned a formal inquiry (the Tooke Report), which was published in January 2008 (*http://www.mmcinquiry.org. uk/MMC_FINAL_REPORT_REVD_4jan.pdf*). Some changes to the current structure of postgraduate training are envisaged following this. The main recommendations of the report that are pertinent to postgraduate training in Palliative Medicine are:

1. The content of higher specialty training and the numbers of positions will be informed by dialogue between the Colleges, Deaneries, employers, and medical workforce advisory machinery to allow finer tuning of the nature of the specialist workforce to reflect rapidly evolving technical advances and the locus of care (Recommendation 14).

2. Training implications relating to revisions in postgraduate medical education and training need to be reflected in appropriate staff development as well as job plans and related resources (Recommendation 29).

3. At the end of FY1, doctors will be selected into one of a small (e.g. 4) number of broad based specialty stems: e.g. medical disciplines, surgical disciplines, family medicine, etc. During transition, 'run-through' training could be made available after the first year of Core Medical Training (CMT), for certain

specialties and/or geographies that are less popular than others. Core Medical Training will typically take 3 years and will evolve with time typically to encompass six 6-month positions. Care will be taken during transition to ensure that the curricula already agreed with Postgraduate Medical Education Training Board (PMETB) are delivered and the appropriate knowledge, skills, attitudes, and behaviours are acquired in an appropriately supervised environment (Recommendation 34).

4. Satisfactory completion of assessments of knowledge, skills, attitudes, and behaviours will allow eligibility for

 i. Selection into Staff Grade positions in the relevant broad area

 ii. Selection into Higher Specialist Training

5. Doctors in Higher Specialist Training, in all specialities including general practice, will be known as Specialist Registrars (Recommendation 37).

6. Selection into Higher Specialist Training to the role of Specialist Registrar will be informed by the Royal Colleges working in partnership with the Regulator. The Panel proposes that in due course this will involve assessment of relevant knowledge, skills and aptitudes administered several times a year via National Assessment Centres introduced on a trial basis for highly competitive specialties in the first instance (Recommendation 40).

7. Integrated clinical academic training pathways in all specialties including General Practice should be flexibly interpreted and transfer to and from conventional clinical training pathways facilitated (Recommendation 41).

8. Successful completion of Higher Specialty Training as confirmed by assessments of knowledge, skills and behaviours will lead to a CCT, confirming readiness for independent practice in that specialty at consultant level. Higher specialist exams, where appropriate, administered by the Royal Colleges, may be used to test experience and broader knowledge of the specialty and allow for accreditation of subspecialty expertise. Recruitment to consultant positions may be informed by the extent of experience, by skills suited to enhanced roles, and by subspecialty expertise (Recommendation 43).

Within the existing MMC structure, postgraduate training in Palliative Medicine follows core medial training (CMT), with entry to Palliative Medicine at Specialty Training level 3 (ST3), following a minimum of 2 years CMT (or GP equivalent) and achievement of MRCP or MRCGP. The details can be viewed at *http://www.mmc.nhs.uk/download/What%20is%20changing%20 at%20MMC.pdf*

There are some opportunities for junior doctors to gain experience of Palliative Medicine prior to ST3, which is clearly to be welcomed. These may be in recognized training posts (e.g. Foundation years 1 or 2, as part of CMT or GP training programmes at ST/GP 1 or 2, or in fixed-term specialty training appointments, FTSTAs), or in clinical fellow or 'old' senior house officer posts, that may no longer be recognized for training but provide excellent clinical experience. Developing training posts for Foundation or CMT/GP programmes allows more junior doctors to receive a basic training in Palliative Medicine and widens the profile of the specialty, thereby enabling more junior doctors to be interested and explore options for further careers in Palliative Medicine.

Postgraduate training to become a consultant in Palliative Medicine is a 4-year programme from ST3 following CMT, culminating in the award of the Certificate of Completion of Training (CCT.) Trainees entering at ST3 from GP will need to apply for a Certificate confirming Eligibility of Specialist Registration (CESR) prior to entry onto the Specialty Register.

Postgraduate Medical Education Training Board

Postgraduate Medical Education Training Board (PMETB) is the independent regulatory body responsible for postgraduate medical education and training, ensuring that postgraduate training for doctors is of the highest standard. Its vision is 'to achieve excellence in postgraduate medical education, training, assessment and accreditation throughout the UK to improve the knowledge, skills and experience of doctors and the health and healthcare of patients and the public'. Its obligation is to secure and maintain standards in postgraduate medical education and training in the UK by monitoring training and outcomes through surveys and visits as well as approving all training posts and programmes.

In setting the standards for training, PMETB approves training curricula. In 2007 it approved a revised curriculum for postgraduate training for specialty registrars in Palliative Medicine (available at *http://www.pmetb.org.uk/index.php?id=650*).

In addition, PMETB approves entry onto the Specialist Register from non-training routes (article 14 leading to the award of a Certificate of Equivalent Specialist Registration, CESR); this requires time-consuming attention to detail with a mass of paperwork in order for the board to determine that the applicant has had the level of training and experience required in order to be classified as a specialist.

The MMD inquiry recommends that PMETB should be assimilated in a regulatory structure within General Medical Council (GMC) that oversees the continuum of undergraduate and postgraduate medical education and training, continuing professional development, quality assurance, and enhancement. The greater resources of the GMC would ensure that the improvements that are needed in postgraduate medical education will be achieved more swiftly and efficiently (Recommendation 30).

Deanery

Locally, training is organized by Deaneries, who (to quote London Deanery) 'work to improve the quality of patient care by ensuring the supply of doctors and dentists who are educated, trained and motivated to play their part in a first class modern health service'.

Within Deaneries, postgraduate training is organized at a macro level via Specialty Schools, which liaise with PMETB and the JRCBT to oversee training standards (Palliative Medicine will usually, as a medical specialty, sit within the Medicine Specialty Schools). Local training programmes are co-ordinated and managed via Specialty Training Committees (STC), which will have a chair and training programme director, whose role and responsibilities is to co-ordinate and communicate between Specialist Registrars, the Postgraduate Dean, the Specialty Training Committee, and the Royal College of Physicians (RCP) to ensure quality training.

Joint Royal College Physicians Training Board

The Joint Royal Colleges of Physicians Training Board (JRCPTB) replaces the JCHMT and JCBMT (formally GPT and IMSPEC). The JRCPTB includes Core Medical Training (CMT), Specialty Training, Acute Care Common Stem (ACCS/M), and FTSTAs. It monitors and assesses postgraduate medical training on behalf of the Royal College Physicians and makes recommendations to the PMETB for the award of CCT (which permits specialist registration) for those completing UK specialist training programmes. In addition, the JRCPTB also has the responsibility for making recommendations to the PMETB on applications from doctors for a direct entry in the specialist register. The PMETB (the UK competent authority in this regard) makes the decision, taking account of the JRCPTB's recommendations, as to whether or not the applicant should be entered in the specialist register.

Specialist Advisory Committee

Specialty training in Palliative Medicine for the Royal College Physicians is overseen by the Specialty Advisory Committee (SAC) for Palliative Medicine. The membership of this committee consists of Regional Specialty Advisors (RSAs), who usually have roles within STCs, thus providing a direct link to training. The SAC appoints assessors that undertake penultimate year assessments (PYAs) for trainees in order to externally evaluate their training and provide input to their training requirements for their final year of training.

Regional Specialty Advisors have a major role in overseeing specialty training. They are also able to advise the local Regional Advisor on service matters relevant to the specialty such as consultant job descriptions and Advisory Appointment Committees.

In October 2007, the SAC published new guidelines for assessment of specialist trainees in Palliative Medicine; these are available at *http://www.jrcptb. org.uk/Specialty/Documents/Palliative%20Medicine%20SAC%20Guidance%20 on%20Assessments%20Sept%202007.pdf*

Why have Palliative Medicine training in an acute hospital?

Most training programmes in Palliative Medicine will include at least a year in an acute hospital setting. The specific advantages of these placements include:

1. Learning to transfer generic Palliative Medicine skills to acute hospital setting.
2. Working in an advisory role.
3. Clinical assessments from early in clinical pathway, when diagnosis and/or management plan may remain uncertain.
4. Increased exposure to patients with non-malignant disease.
5. Opportunity to work alongside with cancer specialists and see specialist treatments delivered.
6. Learning to work with other teams/specialists whose primary focus is not a palliative approach, offering fantastic opportunities to develop negotiation and communication skills.
7. Assessing and working out initial management programmes for emergencies in palliative care, e.g. in Accident and Emergency.
8. Frequent opportunities to develop teaching skills, to both undergraduates and postgraduates.
9. In teams with academic links, opportunities to develop research ideas or to become involved in research programmes.
10. Most acute hospitals have well-established training programmes for junior doctors that can be easily accessed, e.g. our SpRs all attend generic management, teaching, and presentation skills courses.

Advantages of being a training unit

1. Fresh, young blood, rotating through the organization, enabling development of new ideas and sharing of good practice.
2. Up-to-date practice encouraged by training roles and responsibilities.

3. Rewarding personally and professionally for the trainers.

4. Ideally helping junior doctors acquire basic Palliative Medicine skills.

5. Opportunities for participating in research.

6. Networking with consultant colleagues via STC.

Disadvantages of being a training unit

1. Can be disruptive to the team, with frequent rotation of junior medical staff, particularly if there are more regular changes caused by trainees moving early necessitating locum appointments or unfilled training slots.

2. Trainees are not 'service animals', they have training needs, including formal study time (may be flexible or include structured study such as towards Masters' degrees).

3. Time – being an educational supervisor is extremely time consuming (e.g. supervision, undertaking assessments, appraisal, mentoring, in addition to keeping up to date with training issues and attending relevant meetings).

Funding and employment issues

Deanery approved training posts may have allocated central funding (at 100% mid-point on the specialty registrar pay scale); this does not include on-call supplements that need to be funded locally.

Additional training numbers (national training numbers or NTNs) may also become available without central funding. In these situations, organizations can apply for these numbers with the understanding that posts are funded for a minimum of 4 years, but there is no guarantee of pick up funding from Deaneries.

In some regions, e.g. London, all trainees are employed by a one 'lead' NHS Trust to enable continuity of NHS Terms and Conditions of Service, as the trainees will in practice move between NHS units and the voluntary sector throughout their training programme. Where this applies, trainees have local honorary contracts as they move between training units. Study leave is usually funded via the employing Trust or organization (from allocations from Deaneries); in practice in recent years many organizations have cut down on study leave allocations, due to shortfalls in funding.

Getting posts approved for training

New posts or training (either flexible or full-time training) need to be approved by completion of Form B (available via the PMETB website) and signed by the RSA. Although individual posts are no longer approved, only programmes, applications are still required where post holders will be undertaking out-of-programme experience or are training less than full time. Details regarding these processes should be obtained from the Regional Specialty Advisor or a member of the Specialty Training Committee.

Keeping up to date with training issues

Through liaison with Postgraduate Medical Education Centres, there may be possibilities for Foundation year 2 doctors interested in Palliative Medicine to spend time with hospital palliative care teams as 'taster' programmes, possibly in conjunction with other local palliative care services.

Some hospital teams have been able to integrate junior doctor posts into Foundation and Core Medical Training programmes, thereby increasing the number of junior doctors having exposure to and benefiting from some training in Palliative Medicine. For example, at King's we have Foundation year 2 doctors on 4-monthly rotation working in Oncology and Palliative Care. To date, this post has proved very successful with excellent feedback from the junior doctors.

Through liaison with the local STC it may also be possible to be involved in Gateway Days, when there is an opportunity to promote the specialty of Palliative Medicine to interested junior doctors.

Case study: An SpR perspective

As a junior doctor within the National Health Service, you have the opportunity to work in a number of different settings. The Palliative Medicine Specialist Training Programme provides you with a structured but varied experience. This includes experiencing a mixture of the acute hospital and hospice environment. Being both a doctor with training needs, and a service provider in a training unit, has its advantages and disadvantages.

1. Advantages

   i. Opportunity to work alongside senior colleagues who are keen to teach and pass on their knowledge.

   ii. Experience of various units and people, allowing you to develop skills and a style most suited to you.

   iii. Developing professional and personal relationships with colleagues which continue into your future career.

   iv. Opportunity to work with other training doctors in the specialty; sharing and learning from your experiences.

   v. Possibility to get involved in research that is ongoing within the unit.

   vi. Supervision and training of more junior colleagues.

   vii. Teaching of medical students.

   viii. Developing adequate communication skills and techniques to optimize interactions with other specialties.

   ix. Teaching basic palliative medicine to junior doctors in other specialties.

    x. Designated study leave time to develop individual skills and fulfill training needs whilst working towards your CCT.

    xi. Support from your trainer if you run into any professional or personal difficulty.

2. Disadvantages

    i. Training needs may be sidelined if the unit is busy.

    ii. Fulfilling training requirements can be time consuming (lots of paperwork!).

    iii. Repeated rotation may lead to personal disruption.

    iv. May not be thought of as a permanent member of the team.

    v. Limited time to develop working relationships.

Re-validation: issues for the hospital palliative care physician

Following a series of high-profile 'scandals' and the Shipman enquiry, major changes are underway for the process of re-validation and re-certification of clinicians. It is therefore crucial that hospital palliative care clinicians are proactive in preparing a body of evidence that can be used to support re-licensing and specialist recertification. Recent communications from the Royal College of Physicians (RCP) suggests that in preparing for this you should ensure that:

1. You have annual appraisal, using the standard NHS documentation.

2. You participate in multi-source feedback (360-degree assessment) – it has now validated a questionnaire for consultant physicians, the details of which are available at *www.360clinical.com/rcp/*

3. You have a mechanism for logging untoward incidents involving your team and are able to demonstrate action plans in response to these; such data could be used in appraisal as evidence that a doctor is conscientious about patient safety (rather than of poor performance).

4. Your team should be aiming to obtain patient feedback via a patient survey (this is currently a Department of Health Cancer Service Standard); working as a palliative care clinician in a hospital palliative care team it may be extremely difficult to obtain individual feedback (beyond letters and cards), but team feedback can be used to support service development.

5. You should have a mechanism for logging complaints and recording responses and actions to these complaints.

6. You should collate evidence of participation in continuing professional development.

7. A re-licensing examination for Palliative Medicine is under consideration at the RCP (in line with an exit examination at the end of specialist

training), so consultants should keep an eye on the RCP and Association Palliative Medicine websites for further information.

Useful web addresses

1. MMC: *http://www.mmc.nhs.uk*
2. PMETB: *http://www.pmetb.org.uk*
3. JRCPTB: *http://www.jrcptb.org.uk/Pages/default.aspx*
4. RCP: *http://www.rcplondon.ac.uk/*
5. 360-degree appraisal: *www.360clinical.com/rcp/*

Non-medical training issues

There are currently no formal, national training programmes for non-medical palliative care personnel, such as nurse specialists or social workers, although some pockets of good practice do exist with, for example, Clinical Nurse Specialist (CNS) development roles in one part of north London.

Many hospital teams, however, have opportunities for other health and social care professionals to undertake placements, and there are frequent requests for clinicians to spend time with hospital teams as part of their orientation to other roles, both within the acute hospital and to local hospice and community palliative care teams. These placements give opportunities for networking and for an exchange of ideas and good practice, but can be time-intensive for the hospital teams involved. It can therefore be useful to set clear objectives for the visit so that the time can be utilized most effectively and learning outcomes be achieved.

Following initial training courses, which are now University based, a process of registration and re-registration has to be undertaken. Without this, it is not possible for a nurse registration to be maintained on the Nursing and Midwifery Council (NMC) register to practice. To work in the UK all nurses, midwives, and specialist community public health workers must register with the NMC. Practitioners have to renew their registration every 3 years.

In order to maintain registration there is a requirement for nurses to:

1. Complete a Notification of Practice form, every 3 years, declaring that you have met the PREP CPD and PREP standards for registration.
2. Pay the prescribed annual fee.

In order to meet the PREP CPD standards a nurse has to undertake at least five days (35 hours) of learning in the previous 3 years. This can be achieved via any method which maintains and develops competence. Practitioners must also have completed a minimum 450 hours of practice, in each area of practice during 3 years prior to renewal of registration. This is the PREP (practice) standard.

Developing skills towards a specialist post

At the present time there is no prescribed training which nurses need to undertake before embarking on specialist roles. The minimum selection criteria for a Macmillan Clinical Nurse Specialist (CNS) are:

1. A first level nurse registration

2. At least 5 years post registration clinical experience, 2 of which must have been in cancer or palliative care (Note that under UK anti-discrimination law, job descriptions can no longer prescribe a time interval but should instead outline expected competencies.)

3. Normally a degree in either palliative care or oncology

Development opportunities may be available for people who fall just short of this criteria; Macmillan Cancer Relief have a Role Development Programme which is designed for nurses who are recruited into permanent posts but who, at the point of interview, are identified as having development needs to enable them to function at specialist level. It is imperative that candidates possess the appropriate and relevant clinical experience that will support the clinical responsibilities of the specialist nursing post, therefore individualized training and development plans need to be put in place to support learning needs. There are many other courses delivered either as stand alone units or as part of a further qualification that will give potential specialist nurses an increased knowledge base. Information about such courses can be obtained from higher educational institutions.

It is expected that nurses who wish to embark on a career as a Specialist Nurse in Palliative care will undertake specialist preparation and obtain a qualification which can be recorded on a separate part of the NMC register. This qualificaion should be at least at Diploma level, and there is usually an expectation that post holders (or potential post holders) will demonstrate that they are willing to undertake a course of study that will be able to satisfy the requirements of the NMC standards for Specialist Nursing Practice (*www.nmc.org.uk*).

Core competencies for nurses and social care staff

The Skills for Health[1] and Skills for Care[2] programmes have developed a core curriculum for all grades of nursing and social care staff. This will help inform education and training programmes in the future.

[1] *http://www.skillsforhealth.org.uk/.*
[2] *http://www.skillsforcare.org.uk/home/home.aspx.*

Summary

Training future specialists in palliative care can be very rewarding both personally and professionally and increase the standing of the palliative care team within its Trust. However, it is time consuming and cannot be a simple 'add on' to existing work loads. Ensure that senior members of the team have the time, energy, commitment, and skills to undertake the work required.

Chapter 9

Research in the acute trust

Introduction

This chapter aims to give you some ideas of how to start research in an acute Trust setting. It is written primarily for those relatively new to research and for those in an NHS (National Health Service) post who want to resume it. Those fortunate enough to be in formal research training will already have contacts or ideas about how to take studies forward.

The specialty of palliative care needs research. It needs fresh ideas and approaches to the taxing clinical questions that we or, more importantly, our patients face everyday. A specialty has a scientific body of knowledge that is not produced by the work or other specialties.

Advantages and disadvantages of palliative care research in the acute setting

Working in an acute Trust gives you both advantages and disadvantages in trying to complete palliative care research of any kind.

Helpful aspects of working in the acute setting include the following:

1. Every other specialty is doing research and it is seen as a normal, routine activity.

2. The hospital will have an R&D (research and development) department which can at least advise you on the complexities and practicality of getting research done legally and safely.

3. You have a wide range of patients with different illnesses.

4. There is a body of people amongst whom nearly every medical or surgical skill will be found and therefore you can take on a wide spectrum of projects.

Disadvantages include:

1. Many NHS doctor will find it hard to get research time in their job plans.

2. Unless you have inpatients, you will not have patients under your direct care and you will not have specialist palliative care nurses on the

wards; therefore drug and other specialist intervention studies can be problematic.

3. Palliative care research may be considered to be of secondary importance to other research carried out in the larger department of which you are a member.

Before you even embark on research ask yourself an important question – *why do I want to do research?* – Because, wherever you are, it will not be easy to complete and you need to be clear that you have the motivation to see it through.

Why do I want to do research?

We've suggested some possible answers to the questions posed ahead. Many of you will have replies which cross several of these categories.

I am interested in improving clinical practice in palliative care

It has already been said that palliative care won't exist as a separate specialty unless it has its own distinct scientific body of knowledge. We are a relatively new specialty, and not an 'off shoot' from, or development of, another one. Some specialties derived from general medicine already had an obvious way in which they had to extend the boundaries of knowledge, e.g. respiratory medicine, but increasingly medical and surgical specialties have become more and more sub-specialized, dealing with a smaller and smaller range of patients, and this change in clinical practice is reflected in research. Other specialists who see patients with a range of conditions, such as radiology, become sub-specialized at consultant level. In palliative care we've developed in the opposite direction. First, we looked after only terminally ill people with cancer who had severe symptoms. Then we started to see a much broader range of patients with cancer and now palliative care has extended to patients with a range of life-limiting or life-threatening conditions, whatever their diagnosis.

Inevitably palliative care will become sub-specialized and if you want to conduct research, you are much more likely to succeed if you have an area on which you can focus and refine the clinical questions you're asking. However, it may not be most productive for you to narrow your subject too early on in your research career. When you are starting out, it may be better to attach yourself to a unit (or a person) successfully carrying out research in any aspect of palliative care. The first stage is always to learn about methodology. You may have to be a 'distance learner' at least for some of the time as it is much more common for palliative care clinicians to work in units where no one has had advanced research training or experience and where there is no active research going on.

As you complete the preliminaries of your research training, you will often start to discern which areas of clinical practice really interest you as subjects for research and which questions you want to frame.

You want to do research for career advancement

Research is a very tough route to take if getting career advancement is your only motivation. There are probably much easier ways, particularly if you're an NHS clinician. Career advancement would probably be achieved more easily if you:

1. Concentrated on strategic work in your Trust or cancer network for example.
2. Became involved in teaching or the medical school.
3. Participated in Deanery activities.
4. Became a regional specialty advisor.

Arguably the best way, in the long run, to drive your career is to find something that interests you and then make sure that any career advancement accrues from doing a good job and taking something forward that is good for palliative care patients or helps the development of your profession and therefore patient care. This is also very sustaining for you as an individual.

You want some intellectual stimulation

This is an obvious reason for wanting to be involved in research or even for simply writing papers. Research will require so much of your own personal time if you are to do it successfully as an NHS clinician, that there may be easier ways of obtaining intellectual satisfaction if this is the main reason you want to be involved. Alternatives may be to contribute to research studies, joining up with a local academic unit: i.e. being involved but not committed.

A good place to start is to look at the work done by the National Clinical Research Network (NCRN) palliative care Clinical Studies Group (CSG, via the NCRN website *http://www.ncrn.org.uk/*). There are many sub-groups of this CSG and oncology specializing in, for example, psycho-oncology, complementary therapies, pain, breathlessness, cachexia. You may be able to play an active part in one of these sub-groups perhaps helping to develop protocols, recruiting patients, taking part in data analysis, etc. If you are more interested in non-malignant disease, look at the CLRN website (Comprehensive Local Research Networks, *http://ukcrn.org.uk*) as well.

You feel isolated from the clinical advances that are taking part in palliative care

This is a good reason for wanting to get involved with what is going on in the NCRN, one of the research collaboratives or by joining a group which may be starting a systematic review – all of which may possibly lead onto other independent research. It's wonderfully exciting to be involved in research in palliative care and to think of ways to answer the important questions for which you don't think there's sufficient evidence and with which you grapple everyday in your clinical practice. Again, start by looking at the NCRN clinical studies websites; also think about going to an Association of Palliative Medicine Science committee or Doyle Club study day. You could volunteer your services for data collection or literature searching in other groups' or individual's projects. You'll always be popular and needed if you do this effectively, if you are prepared to help with recruitment, and possibly do some of the leg work: you must, however, make sure this a stepping stone for your research career or interest and not a 'dead end'. You could also go on a Cochrane or systematic review course: see *http://www.cochrane.org/* or the University of York which both run suitable courses; other distance learning or short courses are available from, for example, the University of London (London School of Hygiene & Tropical Medicine, *http://www.lshtm.ac.uk/*).

You had a patient whose symptoms were not controlled and it troubles you. You want to find some answers

This is another way that (determined and persistent) people get started in research. Again you may want to look at some of the research work that's already going on, or work towards an MSc, or consider doing a full-scale systematic review and write a paper. A good way to start is to write a case report or a case series on a patient you've seen who had a difficult problem where you may or may not have made a difference. Look at the literature as *systematically as you can in the time you have available*: check whether someone has done a full-scale review already. You may even be able to collaborate with that person or group to take the work further. Substantial systematic reviews should be registered these days to stop duplication of effort (and a proper review is always an effort), but the conclusion in palliative care papers is often that *more research is needed* to answer the question posed in the review.

Whatever the reason that you have decided you want to do research, do not underestimate the time and effort involved and do be prepared to 'play a long game'. You may have to start with a very limited question, project, or review of a small part of a big subject, but better to do this properly and get results and then you may go onto bigger and more detailed work.

One of the most difficult things to do in an NHS post is to be disciplined enough to publish when you make an observation or have an idea that needs discussion based on your own practice. It is easy to let these opportunities slip by, but many important advances have been based on work derived originally from observations made in case reports.

When you start research, it is sensible to be relatively unambitious: do not attempt a full-scale randomized controlled trial (RCT) when the evidence from preliminary work does not exist. Start slowly and carefully within the time you have allocated or which you have carved out.

Research in practice

It is difficult and time consuming to do research for several reasons including:

1. Palliative care studies usually require the co-operation of several clinical teams.
2. Research bureaucracy, including research governance, R&D, and ethics approval processes take a long time. They are there for a good reason but are a barrier to individuals and small groups starting or maintaining research. It is hoped that this whole process will soon be easier, when the single site for ethics and research governance is developed. Keep an eye on National Institute for Health Research website, specifically the pages on the new Coordinated System for gaining NHS Permission (CSP) (*http://www.crncc.nihr.ac.uk/index/clinical/csp.html*).
3. There is usually no time in NHS contracts for research unless you have an established record.
4. The complexity of palliative care research, including the methodology.
5. The expense and complexity of research involving medication and often small effect sizes for individual interventions.
6. The length of time needed to start and complete research projects.

Many of the ways in which research methodology and research governance has been improved in the last few years have also made it much more difficult for those people starting out who want to do a *small project*.

Getting started

If with all these potential discouragements you are still interested, here are some other ideas that may help to get you started.

1. Make it clear at your appraisals and career development meetings that research is something you want to make a part of your career, even if you may not have done much since your student days or training programme.

Do not underestimate the time you will need to give to research, the tedium and frustration of the bureaucracy, and the persistence it will require for you to take a project through to publication.

2. Make sure you do courses and work with departments and people that will start to give you the fundamental skills to carry out research. Make sure you know how to appraise a paper successfully and make sure you keep practising this after any course has ended. Set up a journal club in your own unit if one does not exist. Go and spend some of your study leave going to other research meetings. Try to get to meetings at which research papers are discussed, dissected, and analyzed. You may have to go to another department in the hospital to do this. Make sure you go to the medical 'Grand Rounds' and go to other academic meetings on subjects that interest you or that you think you may want to investigate. For example if you're interested in improving sleep for palliative care patients find out if you can attend an academic sleep unit's research meetings.

3. Buy some books or borrow them from the library on research methodology. Don't buy books that focus too narrowly, e.g. a book that discusses analyzing qualitative methodology in great depth: it may well put you off as you will not understand enough. Some suggested 'first books' are given at the end of this section but, as ever; books and websites are deeply personal choices.

4. You may want to consider doing an MSc at one of the bigger palliative care academic centres; most include one or two compulsory modules on research methodology. If you are interested in developing your research expertise, ensure that the MSc of your choice does include training on research methodology. Some Masters courses will also allow individuals to take 'standalone' modules, enabling you to get some research training to help take forward your own ideas. You'll have to do a small project as part of your MSc or, perhaps even better, investigate whether you can become part of a larger research study. Work done as part of MSc courses can stand as feasibility studies and lead to fully powered funded trials.

5. Keep an eye on the palliative care research collaborative (SuPAC, COMPASS, and CeCo) and NCRN websites (see later) for research fellowships or research training that may come up.

6. Collaborate with colleagues by recruiting patients for existing studies – and ensure that you get involved in Project Advisory Board meetings to begin to understand the complexities of being involved in research projects.

When to start research?

If you are applying for a new career post where you hope to complete some research, there are two ways of approaching the 'research question'.

1. Start as you mean to go on and from the very first day (preferably at the interview) of your job state that you want to carry out research. Ask to negotiate some time for this in your job plan/timetable, or some time when you can legitimately be 'off site' working with a local academic (or a distant but suitable) academic unit. Be clear about how this will benefit the Trust that is paying you, in addition to the wider academic community.

2. Wait until you're established or have got some initiatives going in other areas and then start asking for some time in research. The advantage of this approach is that you will have given something substantial to the organization and they may be keen to support your career development in this way as you are valuable to the organization. The drawback is that you will probably have been drawn into other things and too busy to be able to accomplish research. Again you can always start it by doing a course or doing some research in important clinical area in your hospital. You may even have done a lot of teaching and may be interested in doing some research on the effectiveness of teaching or another educational subject? Or you may want to do some research with an outside body because you have made a name for yourself in particular strategic areas (e.g. end-of-life care). The advantage of this is that the 'outside body' (university department for example or commissioning agency) will bring the research skills you may need (and can then learn at least in part, by working with them), you will be an expert on the area to be researched and the outside agency will be able to bring an outside, rigorous appraisal of the work which you will need for academic credibility so that you are not researching your own clinical service or outcomes by yourself.

Some of the practicalities of research training

Most of the major palliative care academic centres offer MSc courses and some offer diploma courses that can be done part time. You will probably have to spend some of your own money to get any course completed but it is worth exploring options within your Trust for funding:

1. Your own hospital department may offer some money towards MSc courses

2. If you are a nurse or allied health professional (AHP), try to link any study to Trust objectives: if you are interested in the Liverpool Care

Pathway (LCP) and the Trust are interested in improving end-of-life care, you may receive some funding and/or time.

Other considerations

Time Do you have the time to do the research training properly? Of course, it's true that where there's a will there's a way, but you must make sure that you aren't going to take on an MSc course at a time when you're taking on a lot of other commitments, because it will be very demoralizing for you to fail and will not reflect your true aptitude. It may even put you off research, which would be a setback for a specialty that needs everyone to participate in research in one way or another. If there is anything that would make it more difficult to complete the MSc but you still want to go ahead, talk to the course organizer/ tutors to see if they think they can support you before you start. If anything crops up during the course (redundancy, an illness in you or a family member, pregnancy) which will make it difficult for you to meet deadlines, TALK TO YOUR TUTOR.

Be clear what you are taking on Starting research training or research when you are uncertain is likely to be unsuccessful. If you're unsure, *start slow and increase* – that is, start with a low level of involvement and increase slowly. Always, do research with someone who knows more than you if you are a debutant. You will need guidance so that you do not waste time and effort doing something badly that cannot be published because of methodological flaws and does not lead onto anything else. If you are on an MSc course, you are paying for help and guidance and if you have study leave, you will at least get some of the time required done in work time.

Getting started with grants

You will not be able to start your first project by applying to a major charity as a lead researcher for a large grant. Such grants are given to large teams led by experienced researchers, usually affiliated with a major academic centre. It is the old catch of needing experience to get a grant, but finding it difficult in an NHS post to get the experience. Grant giving bodies will want to see that the team applying for money and who are going to carry out research, have the experience, the training, and the track record to be able to do it properly. It would be unethical for them to give large research grants to someone working entirely on their own without the skills within the team to undertake a large study.

Applications to these bodies which come after some years are helped by:

1. **Research training** More commonly it will be expected that this is formal and if you are to be a Principal Investigator, a doctorate (MD of PhD) is becoming essential.

2. **Links to an academic unit** Being affiliated, involved, or attached to an academic unit where you are part of a team or in partnership: you may even be part of a major grant application. Many academic departments are short of clinicians who are embedded day to day in clinical practice – so one way to really use your expertise when starting out is to provide clinical input to studies and advisory boards, so that the research questions remain pertinent to clinical practice.

3. **Completing some research projects** There are various sources of small grants: do not forget your own hospital charities; some of the larger, more established hospitals have quite reasonable grant funds, but they will not support large projects. They are often keen to support projects from 'new' clinicians in posts – nurses, doctors, AHPs, etc. There are a number of small charitable Trusts, with varying remits, which also offer small research grants. Such small studies, carefully done and published, will be the building blocks to your research career (e.g. research done as part of an MSc may be valuable here). Sometimes small bursaries are advertised (e.g. the NAPP bursary) which allow you to visit an academic centre, contribute to their funds, and carry out some small piece of work with them, etc. Keep scanning research websites and your professional journal for particular bequests or funds for certain professions or for certain subjects (see Section 'Useful websites and starter books for research').

4. **Explore research training fellowships** If you are not yet in a senior grade and still in a training grade or in nursing, or an AHP, you may be eligible for a training fellowship. Those published by the Medical Research Council (MRC) need to be supported by a major academic department and need early career planning, but there are others and even at consultant level there are 'mid career awards' and fellowships (e.g. SuPAC grants). There are several palliative care clinicians who have obtained higher degrees with CRUK though sadly these have just been withdrawn.

Key points

Don't ignore other specialist research departments in your hospital and make contact with those doing work in your areas of interest. Perhaps you're interested in heart failure; there are likely to be cardiologists with research track records who may want to look at improving quality of care for their patients with end-stage disease but are unsure about how to go about doing this; neurologists who want to help their patients with advanced neurological disease; and gastroenterologists with concerns on feeding issues, etc. Mutual benefit is possible here.

5. **Start small** A possible way into collaboration is by writing up a case report. It is always courteous and professionally important at least to acknowledge or collaborate with the other physicians when writing up. I advise the latter as you will need them to check the details of the underlying medical problem. They also have the full-time commitment to care for a particular patient. A case report or series might form the basis for larger collaboration or a 'starter project'.

Remember a research project is not only data collection: the time spent in planning the project (including getting R&D and ethics approval), collecting and analyzing the data, and writing up are broadly similar and many people underestimate the time for getting the project to publication. You are likely to have to submit your papers to more than one journal and rewrite and revise submitted articles.

Some authorities (Ian Chalmers of Cochrane, for example) feel that not publishing is unethical and amounts to medical malpractice. You will not have achieved what you set out to do either whether you wanted to further knowledge, improve clinical care or (more selfishly) advanced your career if you do not publish.

Writing for publication is a skill that can be acquired but can be daunting – so if you feel underconfident, search out courses that focus on developing skills in writing for research journals.

Getting a grant

If you get to the stage of applying for a large grant and you are in an NHS post, consider:

1. Accommodation: where will any research associate be housed, consider this and discuss it early, find the money for 'set-up' costs (desks, phone, etc).

2. Clincial governance rules at your hospital: you should have learned all this if you are at this stage but do check and re-check as these rules change all the time. You are likely to have to take projects through your own department's R&D committee as well as the Trust's.

3. Remember: research grants are not there to support clinical services and do not think grant-giving bodies can be misled on this point.

4. If your project involves oncology patients and if it is eligible for NCRN approval (see their website for latest details), you may be able to negotiate using the local clinical trials nurses or may be able to arrange part-funding with your local oncology department. You may be able to arrange to part-fund a nurse who helps your oncology colleagues with projects who are

then able to help with some reciprocal cover for your project. So in other words, you get cover over the whole week which is very important when you're recruiting small numbers of patients and cannot really justify a full-time post but you will also build goodwill in your department. This is still a contentious issue in palliative care as NCRN nurses may not be suitably trained for palliative care research and it may not be easy for them to combine a palliative care project with an oncology project. This will not be an option at all unless your study has been 'badged' by the NCRN.[1]

All the time think of ways you can build collaboration and goodwill with mutually advantageous arrangements.

Pharmaceutical research

From time to time you may be invited to participate in pharmaceutical company-funded research ('pharma'). This will reduce some of the administrative tasks of research as they will usually take care of ethics and clinical governance but obviously you are part of a study designed by someone else.

Some units like to do this as it generates income to fund research personnel to complete their own projects by recruiting a few patients to a major national study.

Other important aspects of research

1. **Research is not something you can do in isolation:** remember to involve people in your department. Consult before you start to ensure that accommodation and time are available and that your research will be acceptable for the department. Does it have excess costs or is extra time needed for seeing patients? This is being increasingly recognized as a barrier to research in the NHS and you may be able to find funding from the CLRN to support the department.

2. **Research is now closely regulated:** have you filled in the necessary permissions and ensured that R&D processes as well as ethics have been followed? Your research will be stopped if you have not followed the regulations and you will not be supported in doing more if you have 'gone it alone' as you will be seen to have behaved unethically.

3. **Research always costs more than you think:** have you allowed monies for advertising costs, computers, desks, tables, printing costs, and licences for

---

[1] Badging refers to a process of approval by the NCRN; one criterion for gaining approval is that the study has been funded by a grant gained in open competition with peer review.

questionnaires – are your travelling costs based on reality or just a wild guess? Have you left enough time for finance to scrutinize your form?

Summary

Remember building research when you are in an NHS post requires

1. A genuine interest in the subject you're investigating; drive, persistence, ingenuity, creativity

2. Collaboration with a team of people who have the skills that you don't have and anything but the smallest project needs a team for it to be completely successfully

3. Intrusion into your personal time and use of some of your money to get the training you need

4. Attention to detail for getting funding, meeting clinical governance requirements, and maintaining paperwork to the required standard. If this is not a skill you have, work with someone who does

Do not forget that as a clinician with a high level of clinical skills and access to patients you will offer the sort of clinical knowledge which the other members of an academic team may not have: you may be the one who has realistic clinical ideas, understand the issues that trouble both patients and clinicians and who can recruit to trials.

Key points

- Research needs teamwork and you could be a key part of the team.
- Research is exciting and satisfying.
- Research is frustrating and laborious.
- You need training to do research well.
- NHS clinicians are ideally placed to ensure that clinically relevant research is carried out.
- Research is essential if patients are to be offered improved palliative care treatments in the future.

Useful websites and starter books for research

E-books

1. *Design of Studies for Medical Research*, David Machin and Michael J. Campbell, Wiley, 2005.

2. *Data Analysis and Presentation Skills*, Jackie Willis, Wiley, 2004.

3. *Clinical Trials: A Practical Guide to Design, Analysis and Reporting*, Duolao Wang and Ameet Bakhai, Remedica, 2006.

4. *Real World Research*, David Robson, Radcliffe Medical Press, 1993.

Websites

1. NCRN:http://www.ncrn.org.uk/

2. MRC:http://www.mrc.ac.uk/index.htm

3. NIHR clinical permissions: http://www.crncc.nihr.ac.uk/index/clinical/csp. html

4. Supportive and palliative care (SuPAC) research collaborative websites (see http://www.mariecurie.org.uk/NR/rdonlyres/27A7D659-6E58-45B2-B312-FE119B1F18D8/0/supac_bg_obj_of_research_collaboratives.pdf for background information)

5. CeCO: http://www.ceco.org.uk/about.php

6. COMPASS: http://www.compasscollaborative.com/

Chapter 10

Personal survival

Why have we included a chapter on personal survival in this book? It is because in spite of the abundant rewards, we think working as a palliative care specialist in an acute Trust has challenges (to use the modern euphemism) all of its own. They are different, rather than less or more than those associated with working in other settings, including hospices.

It is well known that palliative care specialists have significant rates of depressive illness perhaps because of the sorts of people who enter the specialty. We think that there are ways to reduce the chances of serious unhappiness, leading to professional and personal losses, as well as repercussions for family and friends.

What do we mean by survival?

This book is concerned with work and we have concentrated on well-being in that area: we are not focussing on 'self-realization' or personal happiness as an end in itself but rather well-being and effectiveness at work whatever happens to come your way (and it will, 'stuff happens'). Some of the ideas are based on our experience and that of others with whom we have been involved, some on research, some on the general 'well-being' zeitgeist.' There is not room for detailed information on every self-help strategy available so sometimes books and/or courses are recommended for further reading. We also want you to be alert to any potentially dangerous deterioration in your well-being before it affects you and other people (particularly patients in this context) irredeemably.

Survival is an individual quest as everyone has very personal aims in life and different sorts of confidence. You will have to sift out what will work for you and discard that which sets your teeth on edge – but please do consider changing your behaviour or your situation or look for help if things are not going well and take the time to consider new strategies to improve your working well-being. Work is such a big part of our lives that 'feeling good' at work will certainly affect your life overall.

If you go on doing what you have always done, you will get what you have always got – perhaps now is the time to consider another way of doing or looking at things

We will start with pointers to help identify when things are not right and then move onto strategies which may help promote and maintain 'joie de vivre'.

What is going wrong?

Conflict

Differences of opinion are a normal part of life – they can lead to real progress in clinical treatments and in team development when handled well. The existence of disagreement in a team does not mean someone has gone wrong: it becomes a problem when such disagreement

1. Is experienced as a personal attack
2. Feels threatening to those involved
3. Becomes mixed up in a personality clash
4. Affects the functioning of the team, particularly clinical care.

Such events are common enough in all specialities but perhaps are no where felt more personally than in palliative care. Team splits, and how to avoid them or mitigate their impact, are discussed elsewhere (see pp. 67–71), but this chapter is concerned with some strategies to help individuals survive this and the other inevitable wear and tear inflicted by hospital life.

Difficult colleagues

This is one of the most commonly quoted problems in any setting.

First, are you at the stage when you find everyone and everything difficult, effortful, and unrewarding? If so, the chances are that you are experiencing a serious deterioration in your morale. As an extra check to assess whether this is a global deterioration in your well-being or a specific work-related problem, take a moment to identify what is *going well*. If there really is nothing good about your existence, you may well be *depressed*.

Depression is potentially dangerous both personally and professionally. Depression is also eminently treatable and need not become public knowledge.

If you can identify limited areas in your working/personal life that are demoralizing and all else is well, read on. If not talk things over with your GP.

First, remember that you are likely to be someone else's 'difficult colleague'. It is usual not to recognize this difficulty. Use the tactic of distancing (see later), put yourself in your difficult colleague's shoes to try and understand things from their point of view.

Ask yourself:

1. Is it their personality (e.g. grating laugh, embarrassing jokes, miserable persona, arrogance, patronizing manner, certainty of always being right, contempt for palliative care, etc)?

2. Is it what they represent?

3. Do they remind you of someone or something painful?

4. Is it the issue or viewpoint they espouse which inflames you?

If it is personal then you must depersonalize it, (if the person is inside the team see pp. 67–71), if they are outside the team – consider:

1. Analyze the effect they have on you: talking this over with a trusted, level-headed, discreet colleague of appropriate seniority. Ask them to give you feedback on how they perceive the other person and what motivates them: see if you can together find a way of neutralizing their effect on what you are trying to achieve.

2. If you really feel that you need to vent anger, frustration, and personal criticism of the individual, choose carefully *where* and *when* you do this. It may be best to one trusted individual or in an appropriate small group with strict confidentiality boundaries or with a 'personal' mentor. Do not make this a general discussion or a lunch table 'cri de coeur': *you will always regret this.*

3. If you really cannot work with this person, let's call them X, can someone else in the team work with them who does not feel the same way, even if you have to swap or modify project leads or responsibilities slightly? You will then ensure any necessary work is done with them effectively for the common good and minimize chances of a rift in interdepartmental relationships which helps no one, particularly patients.

4. If you do have to deal with X and they are outside the team, minimize contact and scrutinize any written contact you make with them (especially when replying to irritating emails) possibly getting someone else to read them too, so that sarcasm, bitterness, passion, and anger are edited out. Even if they are slighting to you, it does not help if you retaliate.

The indifferent or patronizing colleague

When you work in a hospital at specialist level, it is important to have colleagues who will support you when you try to take initiatives forward within your Trust: without backing from others in your department or other departments you will not be able to innovate and develop. In a hospice it may only be necessary to gain the backing of the hospice Trustees and provided the finances are available (and a fall in the stock market can have devastating consequences) you will be able to forge on ahead within a short time.

In a hospital Trust you will need wider support than that and most of it will have to come from outside the team at managerial level.

Some of your colleagues may have some unhelpful attitudes to specialist palliative care. Some even doubt the need for its existence.

Feeling patronized

Apparently friendly colleagues may radiate an 'I think you're so wonderful' line. This will have no serious support behind it (in other words when the money is distributed, they will not think that it should go to palliative care); surely everyone should be going to the hospice?

Ignorance

Some may be puzzled 'how could anyone work in a specialty like that?' and have very little idea about what you do. They may even see you simply as a conduit through which patients can leave hospital beds and go to the hospice. They will be satisfied with a small heavily overworked team in the Trust.

They may think that anything you do they could do if only they had more time: this is especially true of related specialities such as oncology or care of the elderly. In other words, palliative care is not a specialty at all.

> *'I'm going to take up palliative care when I retire'* Comment from oncologist.

Envy

Some will think that you have far too much money from charitable sources and need no more help. They will think you carry very little in the way of personal stress – 'they are all going to die anyway, aren't they?' – and when feeling hard-pressed themselves will certainly not support your cause, on personal grounds.

Not taking it personally

It can be hard at times to minimize the personal impact of other people's unhelpful attitudes which aren't directed at you, but concerned with personal doubt, fears, or priorities of their own. Concentrate on the greater majority who are pleased and grateful to have a team to help them tackle some of their most difficult clinical issues.

Most of the uninterested do not actively want to harm your department, but they want theirs to flourish and if money is limited and therefore there is a competition for it, they want to win.

1. If you want to feel endlessly loved and appreciated (see later), it's probably better not to work in a hospital.

2. If you want to be able to be immediately understood by the majority and have minimal contact with bureaucracy, it's possibly best not to work in a hospital.

Remember there are major frustrations in working in a hospice, but they are different in kind.

Individuals are usually advised to choose a job they enjoy but when it comes to doing a job to which you are committed but in a number of possible settings, it may be just as well to look at the stresses and difficulties that go along with each situation and decide which of those you find easier to withstand.

The clinical work is likely to be rewarding in every setting

Advice not taken

Another reason why many people find hospital support team work difficult is because very often they're working solely in an *advisory capacity*. They give advice: people may choose to take it or not, they may choose to refer to you or not. In addition when you walk away from the bed unless there's one particular member of staff who's interested in palliative care or if it's a ward where you do a lot of work, you might be the only person the patient sees that day who is working to a palliative care agenda, and the work you have started will not go on when you leave unless you leave very specific instructions. The wards are not staffed to give the priority to communication that we think essential to good care. Acute hospitals are moving towards improving the 'patient experience', and 'end-of-life care' is a national priority in the UK but as we will continually note throughout this book, change in most acute Trusts, particularly big ones, is at that pace of glacial migration, imperceptibly slow. Interestingly people may act on your advice more often than you think.

One of us did an audit on 'advice not taken' at our own hospital and actually found that out of 800 consultations audited, there were only 23 where advice was not acted on immediately and then the slowness was usually due to poor communication within the referring team, rather than disregard for the advice given. It was actually because no one on the ward felt a sense of responsibility about taking forward any advised action for any patient: something for you to take up with your Trust as it is important for the care of every patient.

This is the same for many specialties who consult on patients outside their own environment. You may find many of the same things be taught to the chronic pain and nutrition team, even oncologists when they go and see patients on general medical wards find there is a at least a lag before their advice is acted on (see Section 'Paranoia').

Finding mutual support outside the team

Find mutual support as a team and from outside the team by organizing academic audit or clinical meetings with the like minded and with those under the same pressures. Aspirations to cups of tea/coffee or 'meetings sometime' with someone you pass in the corridor never happen. It is also good to hang such support around facts about clinical care, this helps to depersonalize any slight you may feel at and therefore lower the temperature of any disagreement making conflict less likely.

Recognizing and managing unhelpful emotions

Because of the difficulties of working in an acute Trust it's very easy to let some feelings overwhelm you. We have listed and discussed some difficulties later. They are almost entirely destructive if you let them rule you. That's why they've been given sections on their own. It is not to say these feelings can't actually be helpful as a guide to something you need to change about the way you work or the content of your work but if they direct your actions they will do nothing but harm.

Frustration

In any professional career (in any job) there are frustrations and very few people feel appreciated day in and day out for what they do: think about the arts, trying to get a film project, or play off the ground, for example. Think about politics, teaching, farming, running a shop, or any other small business.

An acute Trust becomes almost a world apart, and medical, nursing, and health service work remains a society all its own with different employment practices and pension provision from other walks of life. Many in the NHS are cut-off from the frustrations that other people outside the NHS have to put up with every day of their lives, it is possible to feel singled out as somehow having a more difficult time than anyone else. You may be, but 9 times out of 10 you're not and one of the things professionals have to learn to deal with is *frustration* without taking it out on colleagues and co-workers. Here from our own experience and that of friends and colleagues are some of the major causes of frustration.

1. You may encounter the idea that palliative care is *solely end-of-life care*. Of course, it is end-of-life care and if we neglect that because it doesn't seem as attractive as other parts of palliative care, we neglect the dying, under-mining the specialty. One may still occasionally hear the view that palliative care is simply about setting up diamorphine syringe drivers and holding hands, being glutinously nice to people without doing anything clinically effective or evidence-based. This is a great frustration and the only way you can counteract that is to know your subject and to act out the different facets of your job, not only clinically (where even wonderful work will take a long time to seep into the general consciousness) but also at strategic meetings within and outside your own trust. It's very easy for palliative care clinicians to get a bit of a siege mentality and only mix with their own spe-cialty. This is not helpful.

2. You may encounter the idea that appointing palliative care clinicians is a *waste of time* as they do not save lives and therefore much better to appoint a surgeon, a nurse on an acute ward, and a physiotherapist to rehabilitate someone, etc. Of course, we do not aim to save lives but some of our actions at the very least prolong happier lives – reducing pain both physical and mental and enabling a more humane and peaceful death with all the spread-ing impact of good on those around the patient which may have positive effects for years to come. We are more and more involved in the care of those with chronic illness helping patients and families to live better and more symptom-free lives, minimizing their use of health services and putting illness back into a social context where patients take responsibility for their health as far as they can.

Positive ways to represent Palliative Medicine

1. You need to be confident and persistent and continue to interact with oth-ers outside your specialty both at meetings and when making the case for a palliative care intervention in the care of an individual patient and family

2. Speaking out when you think you're the only person who can represent palliative care at a large meeting.

3. Continuing to be good-humoured and enthusiastic and championing palliative care initiatives when there seems little interest or understanding of them.

It is essential to remain generally good-humoured (within the limitations of normal human behaviour) and optimistic whatever your vicissitudes. If you get a name for *only* seeing the palliative care interest, giving the impression of feeling unloved and generating the picture of a miserable person living a miserable life, this will not help your cause. People will not help you because they take pity on you, particularly if they there is a 'feel bad' factor associated with your company.

Paranoia

A certain amount of paranoia is quite helpful. For example, the paranoia that a sensitive person can use to be aware of surrounding currents and changes in direction both for patients and families, and, in this context, the health service or Trust. You may be being left out of important decision-making meetings unwittingly. If you find out that it would have been helpful for you to be at a meeting, speak up calmly and confidently, not suddenly and miserably pleading 'why did you leave me out?' If you take that tone, everyone will think actually they were better off excluding you. Taking the approach that your status dictates that you should have been invited will not help either. Assume the 'cock up rather than the conspiracy theory' of how the hospital works.

Occasionally, clinicians are ostracised by their colleagues, or managers may want to get something adopted without going to the trouble of working with or consulting the right people. This is wrong and unhelpful for all in the long run, in these circumstances you need to adopt 'distancing tactics' to the emotion the exclusion generates and not react immediately and emotionally to what is going on or what you think is happening.

1. *Step 1*: Get as much information as you can about the situation from other friends/colleagues in the hospital who may be involved or on that committee or working group.
2. *Step 2*: Take stock perhaps with a trusted colleague. What are you worried about? What will happen if you do not act or are not involved? Who is the most senior person who can give you information and/or support in this situation?
3. *Step 3*: Find out what is going on. If you are concerned, book a meeting ASAP with the most senior person concerned: a personal approach is likely to have the best outcome. Emails can be clumsy or unanswered for any number of reasons and any reply may be difficult to interpret. If you cannot get a meeting ask to book a call. Make further decisions from there.

The most important thing is to try and contain anxiety and make sure you are thinking straight: anxiety is natural but discerning the roots of your disquiet is important. If it is about your status or importance or a personality clash or any other personal concern and that comes through, your case will be weakened.

Concentrate on issues, clinical concerns with patients, and family care at the heart of it.

Sometimes a 'watch and wait' approach is needed after step 2: obey your instincts.

Competitiveness

Competition is not always unhelpful. It's pretty prevalent from an early age in all human beings but competitiveness is present to a greater and lesser extent in individuals. When competitiveness becomes one-upmanship and comes from a lack of confidence rather than perhaps a certain joy in what you're doing, it can be very destructive. As hospice teams know the wrong sort of competition within a unit is corrosive.

> If every specialty can be said to have a besetting sin or foible to which people are most vulnerable, palliative care clinicians are prey to the sorts of competition about who's the most compassionate, who patients confide most in, who patients want to see, who the families keep saying 'are marvellous', who stays latest, who's most unhappy because they're so overworked, who is having the most rotten time because they're the most self-sacrificial person in the team.

In hospitals the terms of the competition are going to be different; who's got most money for their team, who's got the ear of chief executive, who's been asked to give an annual momentous lecture. If you can avoid getting entangled in any of these sorts of competitions, you'll do yourself and your department a great favour; keep getting on with your job-making connections you need to accomplish your work .

This does *not* mean you keep quiet about your team's or department's achievements. Do not forget the hospital newsletter or online information service; these are also ways of publishing important topics in palliative care like the 'end-of-life strategy', for example. Link your department's activities to ways in which it will benefit all patients in the Trust and enhance care for patients moving between the hospital and the community.

Lacking confidence

You may not recognize that a lack of confidence is spoiling things for you: it may have taken a dip without you recognizing it. It can manifest as paranoia or envying others or feeling alone.

Ask yourself these questions:

1. Do I feel that other people look down on me?
2. Do I feel that other people cope with everything better than I do?
3. Do I feel very anxious when I have to stand up and speak up about my specialty?

You may have got to quite an advanced age and been quite successful at attaining personal goals and still lack confidence which stops you enjoying your achievements as much as you should and slows up taking forward new ideas.

Once you have recognized this, it is possible to strengthen yourself and increase your resilience. Here a few ideas:

1. Make sure you are looking after yourself properly (see Section 'Stress busters or aids to personal survival').
2. Get some professional help: from a coach (p.158), or Mentor (p.157), particularly someone empathetic who has insight into the NHS who can help you develop with cognitive or behavioural strategies which can be used over and over again.
3. Improve specific skills, like presentation skills or research skills or whatever you lack for an everyday part of your work.
4. Read a self-help or psychology book or go on a course to get you started and give you ideas about the sort of help that might suit you – dip in to the relevant sections rather than read all the way through.
5. Arrange a seminar/away day on improving team working.
6. Never give up trying to help yourself: even small changes can have a significant impact on improving life and improvement in one area can allow you to distance yourself from something else that is intrusive and difficult.

Here are some books that may be of interest, recommended by people we know or ones we have used ourselves:

1. *Be Your Own Life Coach*, Fiona Harrold, Coronet Books, 2001.
2. *The Seven Habits of Highly Effective People*, Stephen R Covey, Simon & Schuster, 1992.
3. *Manage Your Mind*, Gillian Butler and Tony Hope, OUP, 1995.
4. *All in the Mind? Think Yourself Better*, Dr Brian Roet, Optima, 1987.
5. *Moody to Mellow*, Stephen Palmer and Christine Wilding, 2006.

Envy

Endlessly comparing yourself and the progress of your team with that of others will be terrifically unhelpful particularly if it becomes a significant influence on

what you do and how you do it. Sometimes everything will be going swim-
mingly and projects that you want to undertake, appointments you want to
make will go very well. But an endless cycle of favourable situations and good
fortune are not normal in human existence.

Ask yourself what you most want

How will you judge your team's success? What indicators do you use to remind
you that you are doing your job well? Is it feedback form your patients and
families? Is feedback from your colleagues more important? Is it guidance
from your professional organization and associations (e.g. Royal Colleges,
Association of Palliative Medicine)? Or is it the founding principles for palliative care set out by Cicely Saunders? Is it clinical excellence awards? Being on
the national council for one of your professional bodies?

Try to stick to some long-established, well-tested principles as your guide for
how you're doing professionally (and don't forget your personal life as well),
rather than looking round all the time and seeing which team got the most of
this and who's got the most of that. Inevitably, in the NHS, money and prestige
will follow the prevailing political target or drive. Surgeons will generally have
more money, prestige, and more public understanding of what they do because
the outcomes are the most straightforward and in a payment by 'item of service' world will generally generate the most income for the Trust.

Don't forget that being a surgeon has its own stresses and strains that will
never affect a palliative care physician. In palliative care we are not judged by
'hard outcome measures' (we need some) as individuals where we have to
account for differences from our peers, which can be unnerving but also shows
the value of what you are doing. Find ways to measure the effects of your team
on patient care in your setting.

Reducing stress

Managing and containing personal stress is a professional duty. How you do
this is very personal and something only you can decide but everyone feels
under unpleasant stress, beyond busy exhilaration, at some time(s) in their
lives.

As the word stress has been so used and abused, people often find it difficult
to own up to it. They feel they're taking on the mantle of people who have days
or weeks off work or who work ineffectively for something loosely called 'stress'
without apparent cause. Many feel, as doctors, nurses, and physiotherapist,
they should be in a position to tell other people they're stressed, and not worry
about how to manage it for themselves. Medicine has very slowly to recognize
the importance of stress in health and the ways it affects us as individuals.

Now increasing understanding of the science of psychoneuroimmunology has shown that long-term low level stress can have profound effects on our cardiovascular and other somatic systems. More importantly in the context of work it affects the way we interact with our colleagues.

The stress involved in hospital practice can result from the factors we've outlined earlier and also because we're all human and human events happen to us. Things that originate outside ourselves or events taking place outside our work – getting married; getting divorced; illness of a spouse; illness of a child; money worries; job worries about own or partner's; elderly parents a long way away with illness; and periods of self-doubt, disillusionment, physical illness or depression, anxiety, and onset of a new illness which, of course, is increasingly common as life goes on . A new stress has come with the increasing bureaucratization and of the NHS and different ways of working. Professional stresses like the vagaries of PMETB, investigations by the GMC or the General Nursing Council, re-validation, mistakes, medico-legal problems, and hospital complaints. All these 'thousand natural shocks that flesh is heir to' can lead to personal distress which can at times be overwhelming when you're trying to do a difficult job that brings you everyday into contact with personal distress. Since the difficulties that our patients and families are undergoing are so terrifying and complex when looked at in a clear-eyed way, we often feel our own problems are not worthy, that we're making a fuss about nothing and this in turn can lead to a lowering of our own sense of ourselves which in turn make us feel small for being upset about whatever's a problem for us.

Here are some very basic questions to ask yourself to find out whether you're getting so stressed that you need take active steps to reduce it.

1. Am I losing sleep over this?

2. Am I feeling 'desperate' about what will result if one particular thing happens?

3. Am I very preoccupied with a particular situation or person?

4. Am I having intrusive thoughts or preoccupations about a difficult situation or particular person in the middle of my weekend, evening out, or during important meetings at work on unrelated issues?

5. Am I boring all my friends, relatives, colleagues with why a person or situation is terribly unfair/difficult/outrageous for me?

It's most important to find out if you're clinically depressed, often nothing particularly to do with work but certainly having the potential to affect it. If you allow depression to become serious, it can have devastating effects on your personal and professional life.

Depression is treatable and the earlier the better: if it does not get to the stage of affecting your work, no one else need know about it.

We all know how to diagnose depression in our patients but it can develop insidiously in ourselves and not obviously related to anything or following an event. Ask yourself:

1. Does anything give me pleasure?
2. Am I dreading going to work?
3. Can I concentrate on my work or on things that I enjoy outside?
4. Do I feel I am achieving anything?
5. Does life seem worthwhile?
6. Am I irritable, bad-tempered, unfair on family, friends, and colleagues closest to me?
7. Do I need a drink? Or a drug to help me get through the day or to relax in the evening? How much am I drinking?
8. Are there any habits that I have and I try to conceal from others because I know they are dangerous?
9. Have I lost my appetite? Can I sleep? Do I find myself in tears or have to go and hide somewhere at work because I am so upset?

If the answer to even one of these questions is yes, it is probably a good idea to seek help – even a discussion with your GP (private and off site) may help you to understand whether you need extra professional support.

When you start your job, start a stress management regimen: the techniques you choose may change with time but start one and review periodically if it could be improved and if, because of your personal circumstances, it needs changing.

Stress busters or aids to personal survival

Physical exercise

There is continually emerging evidence on the benefits of exercise. It is good for everybody, whether they have an illness or not and it helps improve morale as well as physical fitness.

If you don't exercise or have fallen out of the habit of being physically active, you may not notice any serious effects for 5, 10, or even 20 years but they will be there, and the longer you leave it, the more difficult it will be to fit it in or make it a regular habit. Physical exercise doesn't have to mean going to a gym, being on a treadmill. There are all kinds of sports and activities that not only give exercise but also produce great pleasure.

You may think you can't fit it in, that so you're simply working too hard or not prioritizing your health. You are a highly trained professional handing out advice to patients about what to do for the best; you should be able to do these basic things yourself.

If you aren't keen on the gym, what about trampolining, tennis, fencing, boxing, dancing, rambling, swimming, or walking a dog everyday so you get the benefits of being in the open air as well as exercise. It's worth researching the difference between resistance exercises and cardio. What about a team game (great companionship as well as shared purpose) or golf, easy to fit in anywhere in the world: may introduce you to other people in the hospital and give you a lifelong friendship.

When you start your job, make sure that you schedule some exercise in your work somewhere along the line and do the simple things. Don't moan about the distance from the car park or the lift being broken; see it as positive opportunity to improve your health. If the traffic in your area makes if feasible what about cycling to work?

When you are exercising (planned or opportunist), remind yourself that you are doing something very positive for your health.

Having fun

You might look at that title aghast – having fun? How can I schedule this in? How can I make this part of beating stress? This is a long-term strategy. If you allow yourself to become depressed, it won't be very easy to have fun until you've done a number of other, more onerous things first but the science of positive psychology and well-being has opened up in recent years and is now recognized that we are able to build resilience (see later) as well as treat psychiatric and/or psychological morbidity.

For too long the only focus has possibly been on treating depression and not on trying to prevent it. There is much to learn about how we can increase our pleasure and enjoyment in life and also our resilience. You are obviously the best person to know how you can have fun but doing something you've always enjoyed is both stimulating and good for our health. It is also helpful to try out new ideas and perhaps if you've taken up a new job in a new town, your old routines have been broken, and you do have to find other ways of enjoying yourself.

Apart from exercise, social contact is good for our health and if you have moved to new environment, *loneliness* may contribute to all the unhelpful things we've mentioned earlier (and stewing in your own juice promotes paranoia and rumination). You have to switch off from work and mix with other people who have no professional interest in what you do: try it; it could be very good for you.

Think about:

1. Joining a club.
2. Learning a new skill.

3. Taking up a new pastime – particularly if its physical.

4. Setting yourself a pleasurable goal (e.g. a marathon if that's your idea of pleasure, a walking holiday, making a quilt, learning pottery, a creative writing course) and taking steps to achieve it. You will then do this in your spare time rather than work.

Well-being interventions

Studies in normal volunteers (i.e. people like you) have shown some very simple well-being interventions, which help focus on the good things that are going on in life may help people not to ruminate on the bad and spiral down into feeling stressed and depressed.

These simple manoeuvres include:

1. Keeping a diary in which you record three goods things that have happened to you during the day. This was done for a week in a study of university students in America were still feeling the benefits 6 months later.

2. Planning to do one enjoyable thing, specifically for yourself each week.

3. Practising meditation techniques such as mindfulness stress reduction (which has an increasingly good research pedigree now).

    Contacts:

    i. Your local Buddhist centre may run mindfulness courses.

    ii. Bangor University runs more advanced teaching and has lots of information on its website.

    iii. There are numerous meditation books, e.g. *Teach Yourself to Meditate* by Derek Harrison, published by Piatkus Books.

    iv. Any books by Jon Kabat-Zinn, the doctor who started mindfulness in the United States.

4. Another technique is hypnosis or self-hypnosis and there are many qualified doctors and psychologists who use self-hypnosis training, which you could learn too. (Hypnosis UK is a good department based at UCL, Hypnosisunituk.com). Learn how to reduce stress and other physical symptoms or to support other forms of life change.

All these techniques rely on the ability to develop an inner focus without distraction from our conscious critical mind and to develop some distance from difficulties and worries. They can be very powerful ways of reducing stress. They can be applied, once learned, at no cost, in any setting (even in the middle of a meeting) at any time, in any place. Such a flexible skill also has the virtue of developing self-efficacy which, we know from many areas of medicine now, improves the management of chronic conditions. There are good systematic reviews of mindfulness based on stress reduction available and we've put one recent paper in there too. You might want to learn about it to consider using it with your patients.

1. Mindfulness-based stress reduction and health benefits: A meta analysis, Paul Grossman, Ludger Niemann, Stefan Schmidt, and Harald Walach, *Journal of Psychosomatic Research*, 57(2004), 34–43.

2. A brief self- administered psychological intervention to improve well being in patients with cancer, Pranathi Ramachandra, Sara Booth, Thirza Pieters, Kalliopi Vrotsou, and Felicia A. Huppert. *Psycho-oncology 2009 e-pub (www. interscience wiley.com)* DOI.10.

Building resilience

If you have a particular problem or distress (and many people in palliative medicine have had a traumatic bereavement of one sort or another which has contributed to their desire to enter the field), you might find it helpful at some point to do some psychological examination of what the work means to you. This doesn't require 25 years of psychotherapy but possibly some brief focused intervention with someone who's 'future directed' or problem solving (this suits the positivist mindset of most clinicians). This information will also help you at work by equipping you with some basic psychological insights that you could later acquire yourself. Alternatively you could find a coach or a mentor.

Self-help books

Self-help books can be very useful. They are very private and very cheap way of getting psychological insights. Some of them, of course, are rubbish and some of them are extraordinarily banal. It's very difficult to advise on self-help books except to say that they may be a good starting point or even enough to help you through a difficult patch. You really have to try one to find out what suits you. A few examples of the most famous or widely read are given in this chapter: we cannot vouch for them personally, but where we can we have made a comment either from personal experience or anecdote.

Professional development

Professional development is an important way of building resilience. The selection of the courses that you need to go on or the private study that you need to do in order to build the skills to do your job as your career development and the health service and your specialty changes is actually very important. You may like to go to the same course every year because you meet the same people but this is unlikely to be a good strategy in the longer run. When it comes to your appraisal, take a long hard look at what you really need to improve on. There are some topics you probably need to update every 3 to 4 years to ensure that you are still doing well at them every 3 to 4 years. These include communication skills and teaching skills. If you go to these outside the palliative care environment, you may find it enormously stimulating for example there's always a 'teaching the teacher' and 'training the trainer' course in your local area. You may also find the ones run by the Royal College of Physicians ('Physicians as Educator') very helpful or the RCN Leadership Course. There's a difference between doing these as part of your routine work and deciding that actually you want to do them because you want to progress perhaps to being a recognized teacher in your area, perhaps working in the Deanery or nursing education or AHPs. There may be no recognized teaching in your specialty in your hospital, perhaps there is very little time given over to study leave. Make some very clear-eyed decisions about what you need to do to do your job better and go and see your head of department about possibly finding some grants/funding to enable you to do this work and *bring something back* to your own department for the investment.

Use the appraisal system also to discuss some self-development that will also benefit your department.

Mentoring

The dictionary definition for mentor would include 'an experienced and trusted counsellor, guiding a less experienced person' in the same profession. Having a mentor, an older, or at least a more experienced consultant in the same or a different specialty who can talk over work-based strategies and actively guide which possible route you should take trying to sort work-based problems is a useful idea for many people at the beginning of their consultant career or when they take on new responsibilities.

A mentor is usually:

1. Unpaid
2. In the same profession
3. Not necessarily the same specialty
4. Of sound reputation
5. Of stable personality

Many mentors these days have had some training perhaps from the Deanery or even from the Trust.

Learning Point: If you are feeling emotionally fragile, vulnerable, or lacking confidence in a major way, don't pour your heart out to a mentor. They may feel like running a mile. If they're sympathetic they will want to help but they won't 'take on' your emotional fragility. Try to maintain professional boundaries and keep the thing as factual and professional as possible. Confide the emotional aspects outside to friends and family or professionally to someone who is psychologically informed or to your coach or 'supervisor'. A mentor will only expect to invest 3 to 4 hours a year supporting you.

Financial relationship

You don't pay a mentor. The 'reward' is a pleasant friendship with a less experienced colleague who is going places and who is suitably appreciative of your efforts. You could buy your mentor lunch from time to time.

Mentors outside the hospital

Advantages:

1. Personal confidentiality easier.
2. Less chance (though not 'no chance') of confiding in someone who knows someone who is part of your problem.
3. Work confidentiality is a problem. The Trust won't expect you to discuss their business outside.
4. Difficulty of access: It's very difficult to meet. There's little time in the working week to meet informally and you won't want to intrude on a mentor's evening or weekend. You won't have much time to travel and may find it difficult to find a private spot for a phone call.

Bad mentors:

1. One who is overinvolved in your problems or concerns and takes an unhealthy interest in what's worrying you.
2. Someone who appears friendly, amusing, and interesting but you gradually perceive he/she is quite competitive and always has to have the last word.
3. One who harps on about the bad things and only considers what's going wrong and doesn't point out what's going right.
4. One who mothers or smothers or who makes you feel reduced – remember the 'feel bad' factor. If you feel bad after you've seen your mentor, change your mentor.
5. If you want to stop, just be busy every time a meeting is suggested. A mentor is likely to be someone with whom it is good to be on polite terms. Don't have a heart to heart about why they are inadequate. With a good mentor it's more likely you'll want to see them more often than they can accommodate. If you feel hounded by your mentor or demoralized at the thought of meeting them, then they're wrong for you. Change quickly.

The APM runs a mentorship scheme. Contact them directly for details. Look out for local courses as mentoring is increasingly recognized as valuable.

Coaching

Think about sport. No serious professional sportsman, no matter how talented, would consider working without a coach these days. A coach may have far less talent at the sport than the person he/she is training but he/she will have other attributes and skills which enable the sportsman to run faster, jump higher, and excel in his/her chosen event.

Life coaching has borrowed the ideas of sport and used some ideas from clinical psychology. Life coaching, based on a sporting model, differs from psychological therapies in the following ways:

1. The person being coached is emotionally functional, i.e. not pathologically anxious or depressed: that person may be uncertain or dissatisfied but they do not need psychological treatment.

2. A coach will tend not to be concerned about where a problem came from, its roots, or associations. Coaches will aim to work with you to find solutions to problems and concentrate on the future, 'where you go from here', not where you have been.

3. A coach will help you work with your strengths and possibly work round or integrate weaknesses.

4. A coach will expect you do to some 'training' in-between sessions.

When you are being you should always feel you are moving forwards and developing strengths.

Where do you find a coach?

You will have to find the coach yourself and it will be a paid professional relationship. You must be absolutely satisfied with the service you get and be comfortable and develop a good rapport with your coach. You have the discretion, and you must change coaches whenever you need. As with mentoring as you develop professionally the sort of coach you will need will also change.

Find a coach by:

1. *Reading self-help books*: if you like the author, there may be contact details at the back. The author may be able to offer you coaching (likely to be very expensive) either singly or in a group. The group is likely to meet a limited number of times and the tenor of the meeting impersonal, but you might prefer that.

2. *Looking at the BMJ careers section*: they often have coaching articles and you may like someone's style. Write to the coach featured. If they are full or unable to help, they may have a colleague who will help.

3. *Looking for courses*: a lot of these courses are given by individuals who run private coaching practices and if you like the session they run go to them.

4. *Advertising*: we are a bit dubious about the *Yellow Pages* approach. You really don't know who you will find but if you look in management journals or use Google, you can look at the individual's websites and see what you think. At least by looking at their website without having to be in contact you get an idea for the feel of the content of what they're going to do, their fees (which everybody finds it embarrassing to discuss!) and what they can offer.

A coach probably isn't for you if:

1. You do have some psychological or psychiatric problems at that moment but they may be useful in the recovery phase to be used alongside psychological treatment.

2. You don't feel you have the confidence to examine another person's ideas critically. A coach isn't a guru – if you don't like their style or think their ideas are dubious, you shouldn't slavishly do what they're suggesting. They're working for you and if you're feeling uncertain of yourself, it may be better at this stage to go to someone who can help you improve your self-confidence and help you develop resilience. *You* are the person who can determine what is the best course of action for you to take and the person most able to discern what will play to your strengths in any situation to help you find solutions.

These list of recommended resources is not exhaustive and it is good (and less expensive) to ask around amongst colleagues (in any specialty), rather than trying something without having any idea of the standard.

1. The Royal College of Physicians runs introductory courses for new consultants and also 'Physicians as Educator' courses. On both of these you will meet colleagues from other specialties and hospitals which is stimulating and supportive in itself.

    i. *http://www.rcplondon.ac.uk*

    ii. *http://www.rcpe.ac.uk*

2. Some recommended books and authors

    i. *Manage Your Mind: The Mental Fitness Guide*, by Gillian Butler and Tony Hope, OUP, 1995.

    ii. *Succeeding as a Hospital Doctor*, Roger Kirby and Tony Mundy, Health Press, 3rd edition.

3. Some recognized authors in this field

    i. Gael Lindenfield

    ii. Phillipa Davies

    iii. Stephen R. Covey

4. Recommended providers of courses
   i. *www.gatehousecourses.com*
   ii. *www.kingsfund.org.uk*

Other undervalued support ideas

1. *Lunch*: there's probably somewhere nice in the hospital to have lunch or if there isn't, there's probably someone who's nice to have lunch with outside your department, nothing to do with you. Just stop and have lunch for lunch's sake. Try and do it once a week.

2. *Friends and colleagues*: utilize your informal support networks – friends and colleagues gained over years of training or practice. Try to meet relatively regularly for a drink or dinner (even if the conversation is never about work!) – these friends and colleagues can be invaluable for discussing difficult issues and for shared learning and experiences.

3. *A short walk around the grounds*: many hospital grounds are now rather like the concrete jungle but you'll be surprised if you explore the territory. You'll probably find some nice 'nook or cranny' or somewhere to sit in the sun or to see a tree! You may even have, if you're lucky, an old-fashioned hospital that's in the middle of town where you can walk to the bakery. Everyone's work is improved by a short bit of exercise during the day – try and fit in something like reading the newspapers or a book and having 10 minutes to yourself. It's often very difficult to find time for lunch but why not *stop* sometimes and go and do something else instead. Remember there's a whole life out there; that's nothing to do with hospital politics, how well or how badly you're doing. Keep a sense of perspective. Remember the patient comes first and the chances are, at specialist level, you're doing the right thing by your patients.

4. *Don't forget the clinical work*: we train to be clinicians, doctors, nurses; we didn't train to be administrators or managers and yet this is a larger and larger part of our job as we go on. As a highly clinically skilled professionals make sure you're seeing patients in a real way, not just dipping in and out of care but really making a difference. Make sure you're having fun with something at work either research or audit or teaching or running some sort of project that's going somewhere, not running into bureaucratic delays. IT'S UP TO YOU! It's up to you to create a good thing at work and not just to feel totally drowned out by the system.

5. *Write it down*: If you are ruminating on an issue: write it down. Your ideas will clarify and you will 'download' it from your mind, and it will become manageable.

Take a break

1. When you go to a conference try and take a few days before or after to see the country or town you are visiting, to look up an old friend. Don't make it a frenzied rush from work to conference to work again.

2. If your finances will stand it and your personal circumstances suit, you may be able to take an unpaid period away from work to do worth thing that interests you or your family.

3. Make time for the things outside work that are important for you, particularly those that build resilience. It is easy to feel in palliative care or the NHS in general that you should be worked into the ground if you are truly good clinician. Actually the Trust and your colleagues and particularly your friends and family are relying on you to do your job but preserve your health so that you not need protracted time off, or get yourself into trouble of one sort or another. Neither the 'system' no the individuals in it will make this expectation clear unless something happens to you. Illnesses physical and psychological are not inevitably the result of stress and over-work but these are potent exacerbators at least and delay recovery. Please do take the unmentioned, unsupported but essential steps needed to survive (preferably thrive) personally and professionally, whatever the pressures to work harder than is good for you.

Summary

We continue to think that hospital palliative care is one of the most varied and interesting specialities with enormous potential for personal interest and enjoyment as well as 'doing good.' However enjoying your career is an active process and at times requires time and effort of will – even in the best teams. This short chapter was written to remind you of that.

Personal survival is crucial to effective working and a skill that you need to cultivate otherwise well-being can disappear without you noticing. Take care of your health considering it in the long term and if you have a dip in your resilience take action early. We hope that you will do more than survive and actually thrive in the hospital environment.

Appendix 1

Referral Proforma

EASTERN SECTOR PALLIATIVE CARE GROUP: REFERRAL FOR SPECIALIST PALLIATIVE CARE SERVICES

Patient Details		Carer Details	
NHS Number		Name of Carer	
Title	Gender M F	Relationship to Patient	
Forename		Carer Tel:	
Surname		Is the patient living alone? Y N	
Age	DOB	Where is the patient presently?	
Address 1		**Involved Professional Details**	
Address 2		PCT HSTH	
Address 3		GP Name	
Post Code	Tel:	GP Surgery	
Ethnicity	Religion	GP Tel	GP Fax
Marital Status	Smoker Y N		
History of Illness		District Nurse	
Diagnosis inc. known metastases		DN Tel DN Fax	
		Community Specialist Nurse	
Is patient aware of diagnosis Y N		SN Tel	SN Fax
Date of diagnosis		Hospital Consultant	
Other medical conditions		Hospital Consultant	
Current Medication (inc dose and frequency)		Hospital Specialist Nurse	
		Referral Information	
		GP aware of referral Y N	
		Date Patient last seen by referrer	
		Relevant Treatments	
Any known allergies?			
		Pacemaker in situ Y N	

PLEASE USE BLOCK CAPITALS AND BLACK INK – THANK YOU

Name:	NHS Number

Reason for referral. Please complete with **all** relevant details as incomplete forms will result in processing delay

.....
....
....
....
....
....
....
....
....
....
....
....
....
....
....
....
....
....
....
....
....
....
....

PLEASE INDICATE SERVICE REQUIRED WITH ✓ AND FAX TO APPROPRIATE NUMBER

Hospital Consultant Out Patient Clinic	**01928 795157**	**ATTACH LETTER PLEASE**	
Warrington Community Palliative Care team	**01925 604269**	**Assessment**	**Info Only**
Halton and St Helens Community Palliative Care Team	**01928 795157**	**Assessment**	**Info Only**
Warrington Hospital Palliative Care Team	**01925 662347**	**Assessment**	**Info Only**
Halton Hospital Palliative Care Team	**01928 753504**	**Assessment**	**Info Only**
St Rocco's Hospice	**01925 630690**	**Inpatient**	**Day care**
Halton Haven Hospice	**01928 701201**	**Inpatient**	**Day care**

Referrer Details	
Printed Name	Designation
Phone number	SIGNATURE Date

OFFICE USE ONLY	
Case sheet number	
Community number	Hospice Number
Date Referral Received	Date of Initial Contact

Appendix 2

MDM Proforma

PALLIATIVE CARE TEAM MULTIDISCIPLINARY TEAM MEETING

MDM Date:

Patient Name:	Ward:
Patient Number:	Palliative Care Team Key Worker:
Date of Birth:	

Diagnosis:

Current Issues:	Action Plan:	By Whom:
Physical:	Physical:	
Psychological:	Psychological:	
Social:	Social:	
Spiritual:	Spiritual:	
Information needs:	Information needs:	
Carer Concerns:	Carer Concerns	

Information leaflet given ☐   Copy of clinical correspondence to patient ☐

If you have any questions and wish to contact the Palliative Care Team:
- Monday-Friday 9am to 5pm: Please bleep key worker or call extension [ ]
- At all other time please contact the palliative care doctor on call via switchboard.

Index